Cupping Therapy

Unlocking the Ancient Secrets

Mei Lin Zhang

Xspurts.com

A New Zealand Designed Product

Other Versions Available

Why limit yourself to just one format?

This book is now available in physical, digital, and audiobook options.

Choose the way you love to read and dive into the story today. You won't regret it!

Digital ISBN: 9781776968138
Physical ISBN: 9781776968121
Audio ISBN:

To obtain a different format of this book at a discounted price, please get in touch with us at:

http://isbn.xspurts.com/

Contents

Have Questions / Comments?

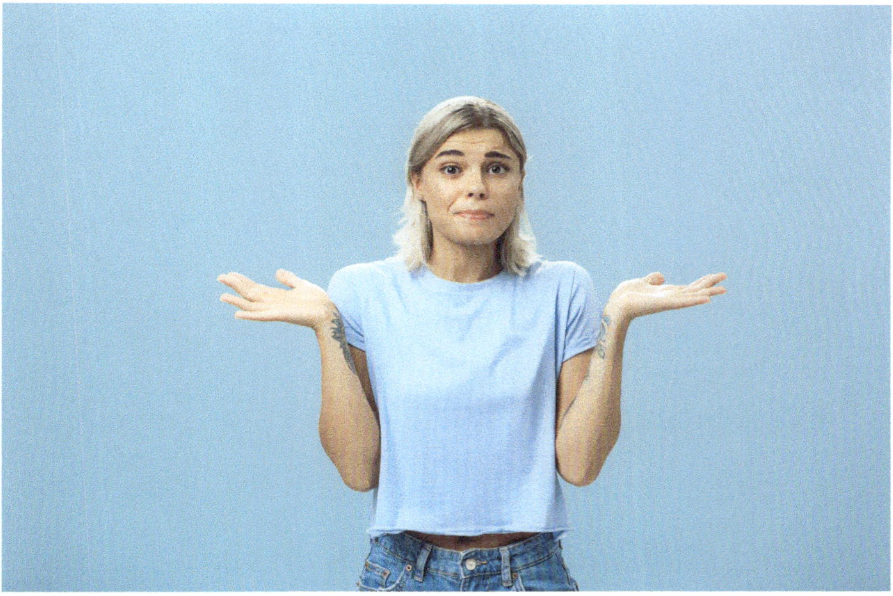

This book was designed to cover as much information as possible, but I know I have probably missed something, or some new amazing discovery has just come out.

If you notice something missing or have a question that I failed to answer, please get in touch and let me know. If I can, I will email you an answer and also update the book so others can also benefit from it.

Thanks For Being Awesome :)

Submit Your Questions / Comments At:

https://questions.xspurts.com

Get Free Stuff

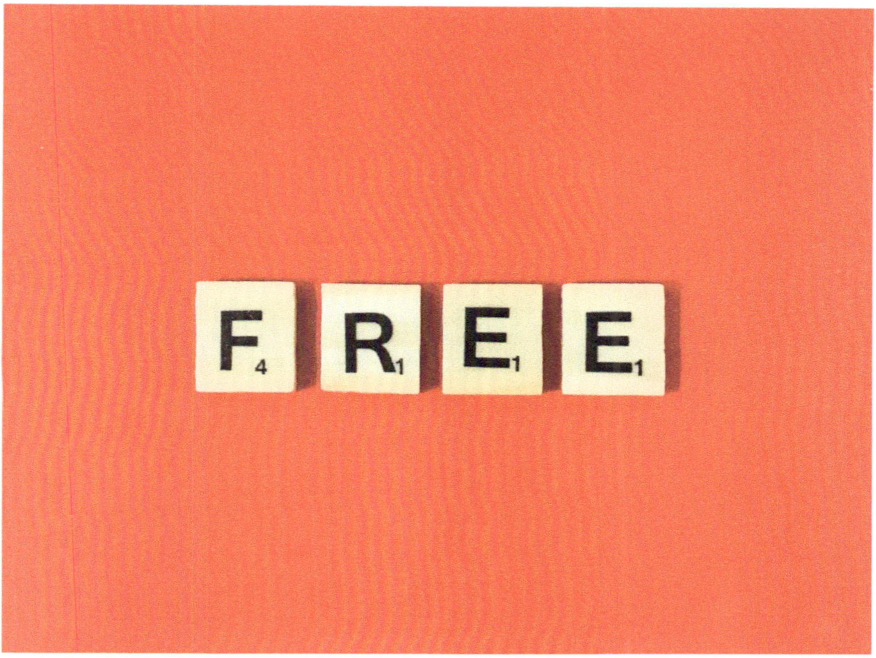

We love writing and have produced a huge number of books.

For being one of our amazing readers, we would love to offer you more books we have created, 100% free.

To claim this limited time special offer, simply go to the site below and enter your name and email address.

You will then receive loads (as we love our readers so much :) of our great books, content and audio direct to your email account, 100% free!

Get Loads of FREE Stuff at:

https://free.xspurts.com

Chapter One

What is Cupping Therapy?

Cupping therapy is an ancient alternative medicine practice that has gained popularity in recent years due to its potential health benefits. This therapeutic technique involves placing cups on the skin to create suction, which is believed to promote healing and alleviate various ailments. The cups used in cupping therapy can be made of glass, bamboo, or silicone, and the suction can be achieved through different methods, such as heat or mechanical pumps. While cupping therapy has been practiced for centuries in different cultures, its modern applications and benefits continue to be explored and studied.

One of the primary purposes of cupping therapy is to improve blood circulation in the body. When the cups are placed on the skin, the suction created pulls the skin and underlying tissues upward. This suction causes the blood vessels to expand, increasing blood flow to the treated area. Improved blood circulation can help deliver oxygen and nutrients to the tissues, promote the removal of waste products, and enhance the body's natural healing process.

Cupping therapy is also believed to help alleviate muscle pain and tension. The suction applied to the skin can help loosen tight muscles and promote relaxation. It is commonly used to treat conditions such as back pain, neck and shoulder tension, and sports-related injuries. Many athletes have turned to cupping therapy to help speed up recovery and reduce muscle soreness after intense physical activity.

Furthermore, cupping therapy is thought to have detoxifying effects on the body. The suction created by the cups can help stimulate the lymphatic system, which is responsible for removing toxins and waste from the body. By improving lymphatic drainage, cupping therapy may help enhance the body's detoxification processes and support overall well-being.

In addition to its physical benefits, cupping therapy is also known for its potential effects on mental health. The relaxation and increased blood flow achieved through cupping can have a calming and soothing effect on the nervous system. Many individuals report feeling a sense of deep relaxation and reduced stress after a cupping session. Some even consider it a form of self-care and use it as a means to unwind and promote emotional well-being.

It is important to note that cupping therapy is generally considered safe when performed by trained professionals. However, it may not be suitable for everyone. People with certain medical conditions, such as skin infections, bleeding disorders, or pregnancy, should consult with their healthcare provider before undergoing cupping therapy.

Chapter Two

History of Cupping Therapy

The history of cupping therapy can be traced back thousands of years, with its origins rooted in ancient civilizations across various regions of the world. This traditional healing practice has evolved over time, adapting to different cultures and gaining recognition for its potential health benefits.

The earliest recorded evidence of cupping therapy dates back to ancient Egypt, where it was used as a therapeutic modality around 1,550 B.C. Egyptian hieroglyphics depict cupping being performed on individuals to treat various ailments. It was believed that cupping could draw out evil spirits and promote healing.

Cupping therapy also has a long history in traditional Chinese medicine. The ancient Chinese text, "The Yellow Emperor's Classic of Internal Medicine," written around 300 B.C., discusses cupping as a method to treat a wide range of conditions. In Chinese medicine, cupping is based on the principle of balancing the body's energy or "qi." By creating suction on specific points or meridians, cupping aims to restore the flow of qi and restore health.

Throughout history, cupping therapy has been practiced in different forms across diverse cultures. In ancient Greece, the renowned physician Hippocrates used cupping to treat various diseases and injuries. Greek scholars like Galen and Pliny the Elder also wrote about the benefits of cupping in their medical texts.

During the Islamic Golden Age, cupping therapy flourished as Muslim scholars embraced and expanded upon the knowledge inherited from ancient civilizations. The Persian physician Avicenna mentioned cupping in his famous medical encyclopedia, "The Canon of Medicine," which influenced medical practices in Europe for centuries.

In traditional Arabic medicine, cupping therapy became an integral part of the treatment regimen known as "hijama." It was believed to balance the body's humors and cleanse toxins from the blood. Hijama practitioners used cupping to address a wide range of conditions, from headaches and joint pain to digestive disorders and infertility.

Cupping therapy also found its way into ancient European medical practices. In the Middle Ages, cupping was commonly used to treat conditions such as pneumonia and asthma. It gained popularity among European physicians, and cupping sets made of materials like glass, metal, or animal horns were used.

Over time, cupping therapy gradually faded in popularity with the rise of modern medicine. However, in recent years, there has been a resurgence of interest in this ancient practice. Today, cupping therapy is widely recognized as an alternative therapy and is utilized by many healthcare practitioners around the world.

The modern understanding of cupping therapy combines traditional techniques with contemporary knowledge of anatomy, physiology, and evidence-based medicine. Research studies have explored its potential benefits, and cupping has gained attention in the fields of pain management, sports medicine, and rehabilitation.

Chapter Three

Forms of Cupping Therapy

Cupping therapy encompasses various forms and techniques that have been developed and practiced throughout history. These different forms of cupping therapy provide a range of options for individuals seeking its potential health benefits. From traditional methods to modern adaptations, each form offers its unique approach to this ancient healing practice.

Dry Cupping: Dry cupping is the most common form of cupping therapy. It involves placing cups on the skin to create suction without the use of any additional substances. The cups can be made of glass, bamboo, or silicone, and they are typically heated briefly before being applied to the skin. As the cups cool down, the air inside them contracts, creating suction. This suction draws the skin and underlying tissues upward, promoting increased blood flow and relaxation.

Wet Cupping: Wet cupping, also known as hijama, is a more invasive form of cupping therapy. It involves a two-step process. Initially, dry cupping is performed, creating suction on the skin. Then, small incisions are made on the skin, and the cups are re-applied to draw out a small amount of blood. This technique is based on the belief that it helps remove toxins and promote healing. Wet cupping should only be performed by trained professionals in a sterile environment to ensure safety.

Fire Cupping: Fire cupping is an ancient method that utilizes heat to create the suction necessary for the therapy. In this form, a flame is briefly held inside the cup to heat the air, and then the cup is quickly placed on the skin. As the air cools down, it creates a vacuum effect, pulling the skin into the cup. Fire cupping requires skill and caution to avoid burns, and it is typically performed by experienced practitioners.

Massage Cupping: Massage cupping combines cupping therapy with massage techniques. In this form, oil or lotion is applied to the skin to reduce friction, and then the cups are moved across the skin using gliding or circular motions. This method allows the cups to create suction while the practitioner massages the area, helping to relax muscles and promote blood circulation. Massage cupping is often used for deep tissue massage, sports-related injuries, and reducing muscle tension.

Silicone Cupping: Silicone cupping is a modern adaptation of cupping therapy. Instead of using glass or bamboo cups, silicone cups are used. These cups are flexible and easier to handle, making them popular for self-treatment at home. Silicone cups create suction by squeezing the cup and placing it on the skin, which eliminates the need for heat or pumps. They can be easily applied to different areas of the body and are suitable for those who prefer a gentler form of cupping.

Each form of cupping therapy has its own advantages and considerations. It is essential to consult a trained professional to determine the most suitable method for individual needs and health conditions. While cupping therapy has gained popularity and has potential health benefits, it is important to approach it as a complementary therapy and not a substitute for professional medical care.

Chapter Four

Types of Cupping Therapy

Cupping therapy encompasses a range of types and techniques that have evolved over time. These different types of cupping therapy offer diverse approaches to healing and provide individuals with options to address their specific needs. From traditional methods to modern variations, each type of cupping therapy brings its unique benefits to the table.

Dry Cupping: Dry cupping is the most widely recognized and commonly practiced form of cupping therapy. It involves placing cups on the skin to create suction without the use of any additional substances. The cups, typically made of glass, bamboo, or silicone, are heated briefly before being applied to the skin. As the cups cool down, the air inside contracts, creating suction. Dry cupping promotes blood flow, relaxes muscles, and is commonly used to address pain, inflammation, and tension.

Wet Cupping: Wet cupping, also known as medicinal bleeding or hijama, is a more invasive form of cupping therapy. It involves a two-step process. Initially, dry cupping is performed to create suction on the skin. Then, small incisions are made on the skin, and the cups are re-applied to draw out a small amount of blood. Wet cupping is based on the belief that it helps remove toxins and promote healing. It requires the expertise of trained professionals and is typically performed in a controlled and sterile environment.

Fire Cupping: Fire cupping is an ancient technique that utilizes heat to create suction. In this form of cupping therapy, a flame is briefly held inside the cup to heat the air, after which the cup is quickly placed on the skin. As the air cools down, it creates a vacuum effect, pulling the skin into the cup. Fire cupping requires caution to avoid burns and is commonly used to address pain, muscle tension, and respiratory conditions.

Massage Cupping: Massage cupping combines the benefits of cupping therapy with massage techniques. In this type, oil or lotion is applied to the skin to reduce friction, and then the cups are moved across the skin using gliding or circular motions. Massage cupping allows the cups to create suction while the practitioner simultaneously massages the area. This method helps to relax muscles, promote blood circulation, and alleviate pain. It is commonly used for deep tissue massage, sports-related injuries, and reducing muscle tension.

Flash Cupping: Flash cupping, also known as sliding cupping or moving cupping, involves applying oil or lotion to the skin before placing the cups. Once the cups are in position, they are gently moved across the skin, creating a sliding or gliding motion. This technique is particularly useful for large muscle groups or areas where deeper penetration is desired. Flash cupping helps to stimulate blood circulation, relax muscles, and alleviate pain and stiffness.

Needle Cupping: Needle cupping combines the benefits of cupping therapy with acupuncture. In this type, acupuncture needles are inserted into specific points on the body, and then cups are placed over the needles to create suction. This technique combines the therapeutic effects of both cupping and acupuncture, enhancing the overall treatment. Needle cupping is commonly used to address pain, promote energy flow, and restore balance in the body.

Each type of cupping therapy offers its unique advantages and considerations. It is important to consult a trained professional to determine the most suitable type of cupping therapy for individual needs and health conditions. While cupping therapy has gained popularity and has potential health benefits, it is important to approach it as a complementary therapy and not a substitute for professional medical care.

Chapter Five

Dry Cupping

Dry cupping is a popular and widely practiced form of cupping therapy that has been used for centuries to address a variety of health concerns. This technique involves placing cups on the skin to create suction without the use of any additional substances. Dry cupping is known for its potential benefits in promoting blood circulation, relaxing muscles, and alleviating pain and tension.

The cups used in dry cupping therapy can be made of different materials, including glass, bamboo, or silicone. These cups are typically heated briefly before being applied to the skin. The heating process can be done by inserting a flame into the cup or using warm water or oil. Once heated, the cups are quickly placed on the desired areas of the body, and as the air inside the cup cools down, it creates a vacuum effect that pulls the skin and underlying tissues upward.

One of the primary benefits of dry cupping is its ability to improve blood circulation. The suction created by the cups stimulates the blood vessels, causing them to expand. This expansion increases blood flow to the treated area, delivering oxygen and nutrients while promoting the removal of waste products. Improved blood circulation can help enhance the body's natural healing process and support overall well-being.

Dry cupping is also commonly used to relax muscles and alleviate pain and tension. The suction created by the cups helps to loosen tight muscles and connective tissues. This can be particularly beneficial for individuals experiencing back pain, neck and shoulder tension, or muscle soreness due to physical exertion. The cups can be placed on specific trigger points or along the meridians to target areas of discomfort.

Furthermore, dry cupping is known to have a sedative effect on the nervous system, promoting deep relaxation and reducing stress levels. Many individuals report feeling a sense of calmness and tranquility during and after a dry cupping session. This relaxation response can have a positive impact on mental well-being and contribute to an overall sense of balance and harmony in the body.

Dry cupping therapy is generally considered safe when performed by trained professionals. However, there are certain considerations to keep in mind. People with certain medical conditions, such as skin infections, bleeding disorders, or pregnancy, should consult with their healthcare provider before undergoing dry cupping therapy. Additionally, it is important to ensure that the cups used are clean and sterile to prevent any risk of infection.

Chapter Six

Wet Cupping

Wet cupping, also known as medicinal bleeding or hijama, is an ancient and somewhat more invasive form of cupping therapy that has been practiced for centuries in various cultures. This technique involves a two-step process that combines elements of dry cupping with controlled bloodletting. Wet cupping is believed to promote healing by removing toxins from the body and balancing the flow of energy.

The wet cupping process begins with dry cupping. Cups, typically made of glass, bamboo, or silicone, are applied to the skin to create suction. The cups are usually heated briefly before being placed on the skin to enhance the therapeutic effect. Once the cups are attached, they remain in place for a few minutes, allowing the suction to draw stagnant blood and energy to the surface.

After the initial dry cupping phase, small incisions are made on the skin using a sterile lancet or a specialized tool. The cups are then reapplied to the same areas, allowing controlled bloodletting to occur. The combination of suction and blood release is believed to help remove impurities and promote the body's natural healing mechanisms.

Wet cupping is rooted in the concept of "bad blood" or toxic substances that are thought to accumulate in the body. Proponents of wet cupping believe that the release of small amounts of blood during the therapy can help eliminate these toxins and restore balance and harmony. It is believed that wet cupping can be effective in addressing a wide range of conditions, including chronic pain, skin disorders, digestive issues, and respiratory ailments.

The process of wet cupping requires the expertise of trained professionals to ensure safety and effectiveness. Practitioners must adhere to strict hygiene standards, including using sterile instruments and disposing of used equipment appropriately. Individuals considering wet cupping should consult with a qualified practitioner and disclose any medical conditions or medications they are taking to avoid potential complications.

While wet cupping has been practiced for centuries, its scientific evidence and acceptance in modern medicine remain limited. Some studies suggest that wet cupping may have potential benefits, such as reducing pain and inflammation, but more research is needed to establish its efficacy and mechanisms of action.

It is important to note that wet cupping may not be suitable for everyone. Individuals with bleeding disorders, skin infections, or a history of adverse reactions to bloodletting should avoid wet cupping. Pregnant women and individuals with compromised immune systems should also refrain from this therapy.

Chapter Seven

Fire Cupping

Fire cupping is an ancient form of cupping therapy that utilizes heat to create suction on the skin. This technique, dating back thousands of years, has been practiced in various cultures and is known for its potential health benefits. Fire cupping involves briefly heating the air inside a cup before placing it on the skin, creating a vacuum effect that draws the skin and underlying tissues upward.

Traditionally, fire cupping involved using a flame to heat the air inside the cup. The practitioner would hold a flame, such as a cotton ball soaked in alcohol, inside the cup to heat the air and then quickly place the cup on the desired area of the body. As the air inside the cup cools down, it contracts, creating suction on the skin. The cups are usually left in place for a few minutes before they are removed.

However, it is important to note that the use of an open flame for fire cupping can pose a risk of burns and other hazards. In modern practice, fire cupping is often performed using cups with built-in heat sources or by briefly exposing the cup to a flame before applying it to the skin. This reduces the risk of burns while still achieving the desired suction effect.

Fire cupping is believed to promote blood circulation, relax muscles, and alleviate pain and tension. The suction created by the cups stimulates the blood vessels, causing them to expand. This increased blood flow can enhance oxygen and nutrient delivery to the tissues and promote the removal of waste products. Fire cupping is commonly used to address conditions such as back pain, muscle tightness, respiratory issues, and even skin disorders.

Beyond its physical benefits, fire cupping is also known for its potential effects on the energy flow in the body. According to traditional Chinese medicine, cupping helps to balance the flow of Qi (life force energy) in the body. By creating suction on specific acupoints or meridians, fire cupping is believed to restore harmony and promote overall well-being.

Fire cupping should only be performed by trained professionals to ensure safety and efficacy. The practitioner needs to have a good understanding of the technique, the appropriate cupping equipment, and proper hygiene practices. Individuals interested in fire cupping should seek out qualified practitioners who can provide a safe and controlled environment for the therapy.

It is important to note that fire cupping may not be suitable for everyone. Individuals with certain medical conditions, such as skin infections, bleeding disorders, or pregnancy, should consult with their healthcare provider before undergoing fire cupping therapy. Additionally, caution should be exercised to avoid burns or other adverse effects.

Chapter Eight

Moving Cupping

Moving cupping, also known as sliding cupping or flash cupping, is a form of cupping therapy that combines the benefits of cupping with massage techniques. This technique involves placing cups on the skin and then moving them across the surface, creating a gliding or sliding motion. Moving cupping offers a unique approach to promoting blood circulation, relieving muscle tension, and addressing various health concerns.

To perform moving cupping, oil or lotion is applied to the skin before placing the cups. The cups, typically made of glass, silicone, or plastic, are then placed on the oiled skin. Instead of leaving the cups stationary, the practitioner uses their hands to glide or slide the cups across the area being treated. This sliding motion creates a massage-like effect while maintaining the suction and promoting the movement of stagnant blood and energy.

Moving cupping is particularly beneficial for addressing large muscle groups or areas where deeper penetration is desired. The gliding motion helps to stimulate blood circulation, relax muscles, and alleviate pain and stiffness. It is often used to treat conditions such as back pain, shoulder and neck tension, sports-related injuries, and muscular imbalances.

This form of cupping therapy offers a range of advantages. The sliding motion of the cups allows for a broader coverage of the treated area, reaching multiple muscles and muscle fibers. It provides a deep tissue massage effect, promoting the release of muscle tension and promoting relaxation. The combination of cupping and massage techniques in moving cupping enhances the therapeutic benefits and can lead to increased overall well-being.

Moving cupping also offers the advantage of versatility. The cups can be adjusted and positioned to target specific areas or acupoints along the body's meridians. This allows for a more targeted and customized treatment approach, addressing individual needs and concerns. Additionally, the intensity and pressure of the sliding motion can be adjusted according to the client's comfort level and desired therapeutic effect.

It is important to note that moving cupping should be performed by trained professionals to ensure safety and effectiveness. Practitioners should have a good understanding of the technique, proper cupping equipment, and massage techniques. Hygiene standards and safety precautions should be followed to minimize the risk of infection or other complications.

Individuals seeking moving cupping therapy should communicate their medical history and any specific concerns to the practitioner. This information will help guide the treatment and ensure that it is tailored to the individual's needs and health conditions. Moving cupping is generally safe for most individuals, but certain contraindications, such as open wounds, skin infections, or pregnancy, should be considered.

Chapter Nine

Cupping Therapy Techniques

Cupping therapy encompasses various techniques that have been developed and practiced over time. These techniques offer different approaches to applying cups and creating suction on the skin, each with its own benefits and considerations. From traditional methods to modern adaptations, cupping therapy techniques provide individuals with options to address their specific needs and preferences.

Traditional Cupping: Traditional cupping involves the use of glass, bamboo, or silicone cups that are placed on the skin to create suction. The cups can be heated using a flame or warm water before being applied to the skin. Once the cups are in place, the air inside them cools down, creating a vacuum effect that pulls the skin and underlying tissues upward. Traditional cupping is known for its potential benefits in promoting blood circulation, relaxing muscles, and addressing pain and tension.

Stationary Cupping: Stationary cupping is the most common and straightforward technique in cupping therapy. In this technique, the cups are placed on specific areas of the body and left in place for a predetermined amount of time, typically between 5 and 15 minutes. The stationary cups create suction and remain fixed, allowing the therapeutic effects of increased blood flow and relaxation to take place. Stationary cupping is often used for general wellness, muscle tension, and localized pain relief.

Massage Cupping: Massage cupping combines the benefits of cupping therapy with massage techniques. In this technique, oil or lotion is applied to the skin, and the cups are moved across the surface using gliding or circular motions. The cups create suction while the practitioner simultaneously massages the area, promoting deeper muscle relaxation and increased blood circulation. Massage cupping is commonly used for deep tissue massage, sports-related injuries, and reducing muscle tension and knots.

Flash Cupping: Flash cupping, also known as sliding cupping or moving cupping, involves placing cups on the skin and sliding them across the surface. This technique combines the benefits of cupping therapy and massage. The cups are first placed on the oiled skin, and then the practitioner moves them in a gliding motion, covering larger areas. Flash cupping allows for a broader coverage of muscles and helps stimulate blood circulation, relieve muscle tension, and address tightness in the body.

Wet Cupping: Wet cupping, also known as medicinal bleeding or hijama, involves a two-step process that combines elements of cupping therapy with controlled bloodletting. Initially, dry cupping is performed to create suction on the skin. Then, small incisions are made on the skin, and the cups are reapplied to draw out a small amount of blood. Wet cupping is believed to help remove toxins from the body and restore balance. It is important to note that wet cupping should only be performed by trained professionals in a sterile environment to ensure safety.

It is important to consult a trained professional to determine the most suitable cupping therapy technique for individual needs and health conditions. While cupping therapy has gained popularity and has potential health benefits, it is essential to approach it as a complementary therapy and not a substitute for professional medical care.

Chapter Ten

Traditional Chinese Medicine Techniques

Traditional Chinese Medicine (TCM) is a holistic healing system that has been practiced for thousands of years. It encompasses various techniques and modalities, including cupping therapy, which is widely used in TCM to promote health and well-being. TCM techniques, rooted in ancient Chinese philosophy, offer a unique approach to understanding and treating the body.

Cupping Therapy: Cupping therapy is a prominent technique within TCM. It involves placing cups on the skin to create suction, promoting blood circulation and addressing imbalances in the body's energy flow, known as Qi. Cupping is believed to remove stagnation, toxins, and excess heat from the body, restoring balance and promoting the body's natural healing process. Different cupping techniques, such as stationary cupping and moving cupping, are used to address specific conditions and imbalances.

Acupuncture: Acupuncture is perhaps the most well-known technique of TCM. It involves the insertion of thin, sterile needles into specific points on the body to stimulate energy flow along meridians. According to TCM theory, these meridians correspond to different organs and bodily functions. By balancing the flow of Qi through acupuncture, TCM practitioners aim to restore health and treat various conditions, including pain, digestive disorders, and emotional imbalances.

Herbal Medicine: Herbal medicine is an integral part of TCM and involves the use of natural substances, such as plants, roots, and minerals, to address imbalances in the body. TCM herbal formulas are carefully prescribed based on an individual's unique pattern of symptoms and constitution. Herbal medicine aims to restore harmony and balance within the body, treating the root cause of the condition rather than just its symptoms.

Tui Na Massage: Tui Na is a form of Chinese therapeutic massage that focuses on stimulating energy flow and promoting balance in the body. Tui Na practitioners use various techniques, including kneading, pressing, and stretching, to manipulate the body's soft tissues and acupoints. Tui Na massage is commonly used to alleviate musculoskeletal pain, improve circulation, and promote relaxation.

Qigong: Qigong combines movement, breath control, and meditation to cultivate and balance Qi, or vital energy, in the body. It involves gentle exercises, postures, and mental focus to promote overall well-being. Qigong practices are diverse and can range from dynamic movements to still meditation. Regular practice of Qigong is believed to enhance energy flow, reduce stress, and support physical and mental health.

Dietary Therapy: TCM also emphasizes the importance of dietary therapy as a means of maintaining balance and promoting health. TCM dietary principles take into account the energetics and properties of foods and their effects on the body. Based on an individual's constitution and specific health concerns, TCM practitioners may recommend specific foods or dietary adjustments to restore balance and support healing.

TCM techniques are often used in combination to address the unique needs of each individual. The focus is on treating the person as a whole rather than simply targeting symptoms. TCM takes into consideration factors such as lifestyle, emotions, and environmental influences when diagnosing and treating imbalances.

While TCM techniques have gained recognition and popularity worldwide, it is important to consult with qualified TCM practitioners to ensure proper diagnosis and treatment. TCM techniques are based on a deep understanding of Chinese philosophy and require extensive training and experience to be applied effectively.

Chapter Eleven

Modern Cupping Techniques

Cupping therapy has evolved over time, and modern techniques have emerged, adapting to the changing needs and preferences of individuals. These modern cupping techniques offer variations and innovations to the traditional practice, incorporating new materials, tools, and approaches. They provide additional options for individuals seeking the potential benefits of cupping therapy in the modern era.

Silicone Cupping: Silicone cupping is a modern adaptation of cupping therapy that has gained popularity in recent years. Instead of using traditional cups made of glass or bamboo, silicone cups are used. These cups are flexible, easy to handle, and can create suction without the need for heat or pumps. Silicone cupping is often preferred for self-treatment at home as it allows individuals to easily apply the cups to different areas of the body.

Vacuum Cupping: Vacuum cupping is a modern technique that utilizes mechanical pumps to create suction on the skin. Instead of relying on heat or the contraction of air, vacuum cupping involves placing cups on the skin and using a handheld pump to create negative pressure. This technique allows for precise control over the level of suction applied to the skin, making it suitable for individuals with specific needs or sensitivities.

Magnetic Cupping: Magnetic cupping combines the benefits of cupping therapy with the use of magnets. Magnetic cups have small magnets embedded within them, and when placed on the skin, the magnets create a magnetic field that interacts with the body's electromagnetic field. This technique is believed to enhance the therapeutic effects of cupping therapy, promoting circulation and balancing energy flow.

Electric Cupping: Electric cupping involves the use of electric suction devices to create the necessary suction on the skin. These devices utilize electric pumps or suction mechanisms to create a vacuum effect. Electric cupping allows for consistent and adjustable suction levels, making it suitable for individuals who prefer a controlled and precise approach to cupping therapy.

Flameless Cupping: Flameless cupping techniques have been developed to address safety concerns associated with using an open flame in traditional fire cupping. Flameless cupping utilizes cups with built-in heat sources that generate the necessary warmth for creating suction. These cups eliminate the risk of burns and provide a safer alternative for practitioners and clients alike.

Facial Cupping: Facial cupping is a modern technique specifically designed for the face and neck area. It utilizes smaller cups that are gentle and provide a milder suction. Facial cupping aims to improve blood circulation, reduce puffiness, promote lymphatic drainage, and enhance the appearance of the skin. This technique is increasingly popular in skincare routines and beauty treatments.

These modern cupping techniques offer flexibility, convenience, and enhanced safety compared to traditional methods. They cater to the preferences and requirements of individuals who seek the potential benefits of cupping therapy in a modern context. However, it is important to note that proper training and guidance are essential to ensure the safe and effective application of these techniques.

Chapter Twelve

Facial Cupping Techniques

Facial cupping is a specialized technique within cupping therapy that is specifically designed for the face and neck area. It has gained popularity in recent years as a non-invasive, natural approach to enhancing the appearance of the skin and promoting overall facial rejuvenation. Facial cupping techniques offer unique benefits and can be an excellent addition to skincare routines.

Facial cupping involves using smaller cups specifically designed for the contours of the face. These cups are typically made of silicone or other flexible materials that provide a gentle suction. The cups create a vacuum effect when placed on the skin, which stimulates blood circulation, promotes lymphatic drainage, and lifts the facial tissues. Let's explore some common facial cupping techniques:

Static Cupping: Static cupping involves placing the cups on specific areas of the face and leaving them in place for a short period. The cups create a gentle suction that helps increase blood flow, oxygenation, and nutrient delivery to the skin. Static cupping can be used on various areas of the face, such as the forehead, cheeks, jawline, and neck, to target specific concerns or promote overall rejuvenation.

Gliding Cupping: Gliding cupping involves moving the cups in a gentle gliding motion across the face. This technique combines the benefits of cupping therapy with a light massage effect. The cups are moved along specific pathways or acupressure points to promote lymphatic drainage, reduce puffiness, and stimulate collagen production. Gliding cupping can be particularly beneficial for reducing the appearance of fine lines and wrinkles.

Circle Cupping: Circle cupping involves creating circular movements with the cups on the skin. The circular motion helps to gently lift the facial tissues, promoting circulation and toning the muscles. Circle cupping can be used around the eyes, cheeks, and jawline to improve skin elasticity, reduce tension, and enhance the overall contour of the face.

Crosshatch Cupping: Crosshatch cupping is a technique where the cups are moved in a crisscross pattern across the face. This technique provides a comprehensive stimulation to the facial tissues, promoting circulation, improving lymphatic drainage, and reducing the appearance of puffiness. Crosshatch cupping is often used for revitalizing dull skin and promoting a radiant complexion.

Facial cupping techniques offer several potential benefits for the skin. The gentle suction created by the cups helps to improve blood circulation, which can enhance the delivery of oxygen and nutrients to the skin cells. This increased blood flow can promote a youthful glow and support the skin's natural healing process. Additionally, facial cupping can stimulate collagen production, improve lymphatic drainage, reduce puffiness, and soften fine lines and wrinkles.

It is important to note that facial cupping should be performed by trained professionals or individuals who have received proper instruction. They can guide you on the appropriate cupping techniques, pressure, and duration for your specific needs. Hygiene is crucial in facial cupping, and it is essential to ensure that the cups and the skin are clean and sanitized.

Facial cupping techniques are generally safe for most individuals, but there are a few considerations to keep in mind. Individuals with sensitive or inflamed skin, active acne breakouts, or skin conditions should avoid facial cupping or consult a skincare professional before proceeding. Pregnant women and individuals with certain health conditions should also consult their healthcare provider.

Chapter Thirteen

Benefits of Cupping Therapy

Cupping therapy is an ancient healing modality that offers a range of potential benefits for individuals seeking alternative and complementary approaches to their health and well-being. This non-invasive technique, rooted in traditional practices, has gained popularity in recent years due to its potential therapeutic effects. Let's explore some of the benefits of cupping therapy:

Improved Blood Circulation: Cupping therapy promotes blood circulation by creating suction on the skin, which causes blood vessels to expand. This increased blood flow enhances oxygen and nutrient delivery to the tissues while aiding in the removal of waste products. Improved circulation can promote healing, reduce inflammation, and support overall health.

Muscle Relaxation: Cupping therapy helps to relax tense muscles and relieve muscle stiffness and soreness. The suction created by the cups draws stagnant blood and lymphatic fluid to the surface, facilitating the removal of metabolic waste and toxins. The release of tension in the muscles can alleviate pain, improve flexibility, and enhance range of motion.

Pain Relief: Cupping therapy is often used to address various types of pain, including musculoskeletal pain, back pain, neck pain, and migraines. The suction created by the cups stimulates the sensory nerves, which can lead to the release of endorphins, the body's natural painkillers. Additionally, cupping therapy may help reduce pain by promoting relaxation and improving blood flow to the affected areas.

Detoxification: Cupping therapy is believed to assist in the elimination of toxins and impurities from the body. The suction created by the cups draws stagnant blood and toxins to the surface, allowing the lymphatic system to flush them out more effectively. This detoxifying effect can contribute to improved overall health and well-being.

Stress Reduction: Cupping therapy has a calming effect on the nervous system, promoting relaxation and reducing stress levels. The sensation of the cups and the overall therapeutic experience can induce a state of deep relaxation, helping to alleviate anxiety and promote mental well-being. The relaxation response triggered by cupping therapy can also improve sleep quality and support stress management.

Immune System Support: Cupping therapy is believed to enhance the functioning of the immune system. By improving blood circulation and lymphatic flow, cupping therapy can help remove pathogens and support the body's defense against illness and infection. This immune-boosting effect can contribute to improved overall health and resilience.

Skin Health: Cupping therapy can also benefit the health and appearance of the skin. The increased blood circulation and lymphatic flow stimulated by cupping therapy can promote a healthy complexion, reduce the appearance of cellulite, and encourage the healing of skin conditions such as acne, eczema, and psoriasis. Additionally, cupping therapy may stimulate collagen production, leading to improved skin tone and elasticity.

It is important to note that cupping therapy should be performed by trained professionals who understand the technique and proper application. This ensures safety and maximizes the potential benefits of the therapy. Cupping therapy is generally well-tolerated, but individuals with certain health conditions, such as bleeding disorders or skin infections, should consult their healthcare provider before undergoing treatment.

Chapter Fourteen

Pain Relief

Pain relief is one of the primary reasons individuals seek out cupping therapy. Cupping therapy has long been recognized as a potential solution for various types of pain, providing a non-invasive and holistic approach to managing discomfort. Whether it's muscle pain, joint pain, or migraines, cupping therapy offers potential benefits that can alleviate pain and enhance overall well-being.

Cupping therapy promotes pain relief through multiple mechanisms. The suction created by the cups stimulates the sensory nerves in the treated area, triggering a response that can help reduce pain. The sensory nerves play a crucial role in transmitting pain signals to the brain. By stimulating these nerves, cupping therapy may disrupt or diminish the pain signals, providing relief.

Furthermore, the suction created by cupping therapy helps to increase blood circulation to the affected area. Improved blood circulation delivers oxygen, nutrients, and immune cells to the tissues, promoting healing and reducing pain. It also aids in the removal of metabolic waste and inflammatory byproducts, contributing to the overall reduction of pain and inflammation.

Cupping therapy is commonly used to address musculoskeletal pain, such as back pain, neck pain, and muscle soreness. The cups are often placed directly over the painful areas or along the affected muscle groups. The suction created by the cups helps to relax tense muscles, release muscle knots, and alleviate muscle stiffness, providing relief from muscular pain.

For individuals suffering from joint pain, cupping therapy can be beneficial as well. By promoting blood circulation and reducing inflammation, cupping therapy can help ease joint pain and stiffness associated with conditions like arthritis. The cups are typically applied around the affected joint, allowing the therapeutic effects to target the specific area and provide relief.

Cupping therapy has also been found to be effective in reducing the frequency and intensity of migraines. By improving blood circulation and promoting relaxation, cupping therapy may help alleviate the symptoms of migraines. The cups are often applied to the neck, upper back, and shoulders, targeting areas commonly associated with tension and migraine triggers.

It is important to note that while cupping therapy offers potential pain relief, it should be used as a complementary therapy and not a substitute for professional medical care. Individuals experiencing chronic or severe pain should consult with a healthcare provider to determine the underlying cause of the pain and develop a comprehensive treatment plan.

Additionally, cupping therapy should be performed by trained professionals to ensure safe and effective treatment. The cups should be applied to clean and sanitized skin to reduce the risk of infection. Individuals with certain health conditions, such as bleeding disorders or skin infections, should consult their healthcare provider before undergoing cupping therapy.

Chapter Fifteen

Improved Blood Circulation

Improved blood circulation is a significant benefit associated with cupping therapy. Cupping therapy, with its unique suction technique, can enhance blood flow throughout the body, supporting overall health and well-being. By promoting circulation, cupping therapy provides a range of potential benefits that contribute to improved physiological function and healing processes.

During cupping therapy, the cups create a vacuum effect on the skin, which leads to the expansion of blood vessels. This expansion, known as vasodilation, allows for increased blood flow to the area being treated. The cups may be placed directly on the skin or moved along specific pathways to target different areas of the body.

As blood flow increases, more oxygen and nutrients are delivered to the tissues. Oxygen is crucial for cellular metabolism, and improved oxygenation promotes cellular function and supports the body's healing processes. Furthermore, the delivery of nutrients aids in tissue repair, maintenance, and overall cellular health.

The enhanced blood circulation achieved through cupping therapy also facilitates the removal of waste products and toxins from the body. As blood flow increases, metabolic waste and toxins are carried away more efficiently, promoting detoxification. This cleansing effect can support organ function, improve cellular health, and contribute to overall well-being.

Cupping therapy's impact on blood circulation can have systemic benefits for the body. By improving circulation, cupping therapy supports cardiovascular health. Enhanced blood flow reduces the workload on the heart, as the heart can pump blood more efficiently throughout the body. This can contribute to better cardiovascular function, helping to maintain healthy blood pressure and reducing the risk of certain cardiovascular conditions.

Improved blood circulation can also have positive effects on the musculoskeletal system. The increased delivery of oxygen and nutrients to muscles, tendons, and ligaments can enhance their function, promote healing, and reduce muscle soreness and stiffness. Cupping therapy is often used to address musculoskeletal pain, such as back pain and muscle tension, as improved blood circulation helps to alleviate discomfort and support the healing process.

In addition to musculoskeletal benefits, cupping therapy's impact on blood circulation can also extend to the skin. The increased blood flow to the skin can promote a healthy complexion and improve skin tone. Nutrients delivered through improved circulation contribute to the nourishment of skin cells, enhancing their vitality and promoting a radiant appearance.

It is important to note that cupping therapy should be performed by trained professionals to ensure safe and effective treatment. The cups should be applied to clean and sanitized skin to minimize the risk of infection. Individuals with certain health conditions, such as bleeding disorders or skin infections, should consult their healthcare provider before undergoing cupping therapy.

While cupping therapy has shown promise in improving blood circulation, it should be used as a complementary therapy and not as a substitute for professional medical care. Individuals with chronic or severe health conditions should consult with healthcare providers to develop comprehensive treatment plans.

Chapter Sixteen

Reduced Inflammation

Reduced inflammation is a significant benefit associated with cupping therapy. Cupping therapy has long been recognized for its potential to alleviate inflammation and support the body's healing processes. By creating suction on the skin, cupping therapy offers a non-invasive approach to addressing inflammation and promoting overall well-being.

Inflammation is a natural immune response triggered by the body to protect against injury, infection, or other harmful stimuli. However, chronic inflammation can contribute to various health conditions and symptoms. Cupping therapy has been found to help reduce inflammation through several mechanisms.

Firstly, cupping therapy promotes blood circulation in the treated areas. The suction created by the cups helps to dilate blood vessels, increasing blood flow to the region. Improved blood circulation brings oxygen and nutrients to the tissues, aiding in the removal of inflammatory byproducts and supporting the body's natural healing processes. By removing stagnant blood and promoting fresh blood flow, cupping therapy can help reduce localized inflammation.

Secondly, cupping therapy affects the lymphatic system, which plays a crucial role in the immune response and inflammation. The suction created by the cups helps to stimulate the flow of lymphatic fluid, enhancing the body's ability to remove toxins and waste products. This can help reduce inflammation by facilitating the drainage of excess fluid and reducing tissue swelling.

Cupping therapy is often used to address conditions associated with inflammation, such as musculoskeletal pain, arthritis, and sports injuries. By reducing inflammation, cupping therapy can alleviate pain, improve joint mobility, and enhance overall comfort. The cups are typically placed over the affected areas, allowing the therapeutic effects to target the specific site of inflammation.

It is important to note that cupping therapy should be performed by trained professionals to ensure safe and effective treatment. The cups should be applied to clean and sanitized skin to minimize the risk of infection. Individuals with certain health conditions, such as bleeding disorders or skin infections, should consult their healthcare provider before undergoing cupping therapy.

In addition to localized inflammation, cupping therapy has shown potential in reducing systemic inflammation. Research suggests that cupping therapy can modulate the immune response and inhibit the production of pro-inflammatory substances. This systemic anti-inflammatory effect may contribute to overall well-being and help manage conditions associated with chronic inflammation, such as autoimmune diseases.

Furthermore, cupping therapy can support the reduction of inflammation-related symptoms. For example, individuals with respiratory conditions, such as asthma or allergies, may experience relief from cupping therapy. The cups are often applied to the back or chest area, stimulating blood flow and lymphatic drainage, which can help reduce inflammation and alleviate respiratory symptoms.

While cupping therapy offers potential benefits in reducing inflammation, it should be used as a complementary therapy and not a substitute for professional medical care. Individuals with chronic or severe health conditions should consult with healthcare providers to develop comprehensive treatment plans.

Chapter Seventeen

Relaxation and Stress Reduction

Relaxation and stress reduction are key benefits associated with cupping therapy. Cupping therapy offers individuals a holistic approach to unwind, de-stress, and promote overall well-being. Through its unique suction technique, cupping therapy induces a state of relaxation and helps alleviate the physical and mental effects of stress.

Cupping therapy promotes relaxation by stimulating the parasympathetic nervous system, which is responsible for the body's rest and digest response. The gentle suction created by the cups triggers a relaxation response in the body, leading to a decrease in heart rate, blood pressure, and muscle tension. This physiological shift allows individuals to enter a more relaxed state, both physically and mentally.

The therapeutic experience of cupping therapy can be deeply soothing and calming. Many individuals find the sensation of the cups on their skin to be comforting and nurturing. The cups are often applied to specific areas of tension or stress, such as the back, neck, or shoulders, allowing the therapeutic effects to target these areas and promote relaxation.

The relaxation induced by cupping therapy has a ripple effect on the mind and body. As the body relaxes, stress hormones, such as cortisol, are reduced, and feel-good hormones, such as endorphins, are released. This hormonal balance contributes to an improved mood, reduced anxiety, and an overall sense of well-being.

Cupping therapy can be particularly beneficial for individuals experiencing stress-related symptoms, such as headaches, migraines, and muscle tension. The cups are often applied to the upper back and neck area, where stress and tension tend to accumulate. The gentle suction helps to release muscle knots and reduce muscle stiffness, providing relief from stress-related discomfort.

Furthermore, cupping therapy offers individuals a mindful and meditative experience. During the therapy session, individuals can focus on their breath and body sensations, allowing them to enter a state of mindfulness. This mindfulness practice can help individuals let go of stress, worries, and mental chatter, promoting a sense of calm and relaxation.

Regular cupping therapy sessions can contribute to long-term stress reduction. By incorporating cupping therapy into a self-care routine, individuals can proactively manage stress levels and promote overall well-being. The relaxation and stress reduction benefits of cupping therapy can have positive impacts on various aspects of life, including sleep quality, mood, and overall resilience to stress.

It is important to note that cupping therapy should be performed by trained professionals to ensure safe and effective treatment. The cups should be applied to clean and sanitized skin to minimize the risk of infection. Individuals with certain health conditions, such as bleeding disorders or skin infections, should consult their healthcare provider before undergoing cupping therapy.

In addition to cupping therapy, individuals can enhance relaxation and stress reduction by incorporating complementary practices. Deep breathing exercises, meditation, and self-care activities, such as taking warm baths or practicing gentle stretching, can complement the benefits of cupping therapy and promote overall relaxation.

Chapter Eighteen

Cupping Therapy for Specific Conditions

Cupping therapy is a versatile treatment modality that can be used to address a wide range of specific conditions. While cupping therapy is often sought after for its general health benefits, it can also be tailored to target specific ailments and promote healing in a targeted manner. Let's explore some specific conditions for which cupping therapy has shown promise:

Musculoskeletal Pain: Cupping therapy is commonly used to alleviate musculoskeletal pain, such as back pain, neck pain, and muscle tension. The cups are applied to the affected areas, creating suction that helps release muscle knots, improve blood circulation, and reduce inflammation. By targeting the source of pain, cupping therapy can provide relief and promote healing.

Sports Injuries: Cupping therapy has gained popularity in the realm of sports medicine as a means to promote recovery and enhance performance. Athletes often seek cupping therapy to address sports-related injuries, such as sprains, strains, and muscle soreness. The therapy helps to improve blood circulation, reduce swelling, and speed up the healing process, allowing athletes to return to their activities more quickly.

Respiratory Conditions: Cupping therapy can provide relief for respiratory conditions such as asthma, bronchitis, and congestion. By applying cups to the back and chest, cupping therapy stimulates blood flow, enhances lymphatic drainage, and promotes the expectoration of mucus. This can help alleviate symptoms, improve breathing, and support respiratory health.

Digestive Disorders: Cupping therapy may be beneficial for individuals with digestive disorders, including gastritis, irritable bowel syndrome (IBS), and constipation. The cups are often applied to the abdominal area, aiding in the relaxation of the digestive muscles and improving blood flow to the gastrointestinal tract. This can help alleviate pain, reduce inflammation, and promote healthy digestion.

Skin Conditions: Cupping therapy can be used to address various skin conditions, such as acne, eczema, and psoriasis. By improving blood circulation and promoting lymphatic drainage, cupping therapy supports the removal of toxins, reduces inflammation, and promotes healing of the skin. The cups can be applied directly to the affected areas or moved along the lymphatic pathways to enhance the therapeutic effects.

Headaches and Migraines: Cupping therapy has shown promise in relieving headaches and migraines. The cups are often applied to the neck, upper back, and shoulders, targeting areas commonly associated with tension and trigger points. The therapy helps to release muscle tension, improve blood circulation, and alleviate pain, providing relief from headache symptoms.

It is important to note that cupping therapy should be performed by trained professionals to ensure safe and effective treatment. The cups should be applied to clean and sanitized skin to minimize the risk of infection. Individuals with certain health conditions, such as bleeding disorders or skin infections, should consult their healthcare provider before undergoing cupping therapy.

Cupping therapy can be used as a standalone treatment or in combination with other modalities to address specific conditions. It is often incorporated into a comprehensive treatment plan that may include lifestyle modifications, dietary changes, and other therapeutic interventions. Working with a healthcare provider or qualified cupping therapist can help determine the best approach for individual needs.

Chapter Nineteen

Cupping Therapy for Back Pain

Cupping therapy has gained recognition as a potential treatment for back pain. Back pain is a common condition that can be caused by various factors, including muscle strain, poor posture, and underlying spinal conditions. Cupping therapy offers a non-invasive and holistic approach to addressing back pain, providing potential benefits for pain relief, muscle relaxation, and overall healing.

When it comes to back pain, cupping therapy targets the affected areas directly. The cups are typically applied to the back, either stationary or in a gliding motion, depending on the practitioner's approach and the individual's specific needs. Let's explore how cupping therapy can be beneficial for back pain:

Pain Relief: Cupping therapy has shown potential in providing pain relief for back pain. The suction created by the cups helps to release muscle tension and alleviate muscle knots, which are common contributors to back pain. By improving blood circulation and promoting the delivery of oxygen and nutrients to the affected area, cupping therapy can help reduce pain and promote the body's natural healing processes.

Muscle Relaxation: Back pain often involves muscle tightness and stiffness. Cupping therapy helps to relax the muscles in the back, releasing tension and promoting muscle flexibility. The cups create a gentle suction that draws blood to the surface, improving blood circulation and stimulating the relaxation response in the muscles. This muscle relaxation can contribute to pain reduction and improve range of motion.

Improved Blood Circulation: Cupping therapy improves blood circulation to the back, which aids in the healing process. The increased blood flow brings oxygen and nutrients to the tissues, supporting the repair of damaged muscles and reducing inflammation. By enhancing blood circulation, cupping therapy can help address the underlying causes of back pain and promote overall healing.

Reduction of Inflammation: Cupping therapy can help reduce inflammation in the back. Inflammation is a common factor in many cases of back pain and can contribute to pain and discomfort. The cups create a suction effect that promotes the drainage of excess fluid and reduces tissue swelling. By reducing inflammation, cupping therapy can alleviate pain and support the healing process.

Complementary Therapy: Cupping therapy can be used as a complementary therapy alongside other treatments for back pain. It can enhance the effects of other modalities such as massage, chiropractic adjustments, and physical therapy. Cupping therapy can be integrated into a comprehensive treatment plan tailored to an individual's specific needs, addressing multiple aspects of back pain management.

It is important to note that cupping therapy should be performed by trained professionals to ensure safe and effective treatment. The cups should be applied to clean and sanitized skin to minimize the risk of infection. Individuals with certain health conditions, such as bleeding disorders or skin infections, should consult their healthcare provider before undergoing cupping therapy.

Chapter Twenty

Cupping Therapy for Migraines and Headaches

Cupping therapy has emerged as a potential treatment for migraines and headaches, offering a holistic and non-invasive approach to address these debilitating conditions. Migraines and headaches can be disruptive to daily life, causing intense pain, sensitivity to light and sound, and overall discomfort. Cupping therapy provides potential benefits for pain relief, muscle relaxation, and overall symptom management.

When it comes to migraines and headaches, cupping therapy is typically applied to the neck, upper back, and shoulders—areas commonly associated with tension and trigger points. The cups can be stationary or moved in a gliding motion, depending on the practitioner's approach and the individual's specific needs. Let's explore how cupping therapy can be beneficial for migraines and headaches:

Pain Relief: Cupping therapy has shown promise in providing relief from migraine and headache pain. The gentle suction created by the cups helps to release muscle tension and alleviate muscle knots in the neck and upper back. By improving blood circulation and promoting the delivery of oxygen and nutrients to the affected area, cupping therapy can help reduce pain and provide relief from migraine and headache symptoms.

Muscle Relaxation: Migraines and headaches are often accompanied by muscle tension in the neck and shoulders. Cupping therapy helps to relax the muscles in these areas, relieving tension and promoting muscle flexibility. The cups create a gentle suction that increases blood flow, stimulates the relaxation response, and aids in muscle relaxation. This muscle relaxation can contribute to pain reduction and alleviate migraine and headache symptoms.

Improved Blood Circulation: Cupping therapy enhances blood circulation in the targeted areas, which can be beneficial for migraines and headaches. The increased blood flow brings oxygen and nutrients to the tissues, supporting the relaxation of blood vessels and reducing the intensity of migraines and headaches. By improving blood circulation, cupping therapy helps address the underlying causes of these conditions and promotes overall symptom management.

Reduction of Trigger Points: Cupping therapy can help address trigger points in the neck and upper back that can contribute to migraines and headaches. Trigger points are tight knots or bands of muscle fibers that can cause pain and referred pain. The suction effect created by the cups helps to release these trigger points, relieving pain and reducing the frequency and intensity of migraines and headaches.

Stress Reduction: Cupping therapy has a calming effect on the nervous system, which can be beneficial for individuals experiencing migraines and headaches triggered or exacerbated by stress. The therapeutic experience of cupping therapy induces relaxation, reduces anxiety, and promotes a sense of well-being. By alleviating stress and promoting relaxation, cupping therapy can contribute to overall migraine and headache management.

It is important to note that cupping therapy should be performed by trained professionals to ensure safe and effective treatment. The cups should be applied to clean and sanitized skin to minimize the risk of infection. Individuals with certain health conditions, such as bleeding disorders or skin infections, should consult their healthcare provider before undergoing cupping therapy.

Chapter Twenty-One

Cupping Therapy for Respiratory Disorders

Cupping therapy has gained recognition as a potential treatment for respiratory disorders, offering a non-invasive and holistic approach to support respiratory health. Respiratory disorders encompass a range of conditions, including asthma, bronchitis, congestion, and allergies. Cupping therapy provides potential benefits for symptom relief, improved breathing, and overall respiratory well-being.

When it comes to respiratory disorders, cupping therapy focuses on the back, chest, and upper respiratory areas. The cups are typically applied in these regions to stimulate blood circulation, enhance lymphatic drainage, and promote expectoration of mucus. Let's explore how cupping therapy can be beneficial for respiratory disorders:

Improved Breathing: Cupping therapy can help individuals with respiratory disorders improve their breathing. By applying cups to the chest and back, cupping therapy stimulates blood flow and lymphatic drainage, which can help reduce congestion and open up the airways. The enhanced circulation and clearance of mucus contribute to improved airflow, making breathing easier for individuals with respiratory disorders.

Reduction of Chest Congestion: Cupping therapy aids in reducing chest congestion, a common symptom in respiratory disorders. The cups create a suction effect that promotes the movement of lymphatic fluid, assisting in the clearance of excess mucus from the lungs and respiratory tract. This can help alleviate coughing, chest tightness, and difficulty in breathing associated with respiratory disorders.

Relaxation of Respiratory Muscles: Cupping therapy can relax the respiratory muscles, helping individuals with respiratory disorders manage their symptoms more effectively. The gentle suction applied to the back and chest stimulates blood circulation and induces a state of relaxation, reducing muscle tension and promoting respiratory muscle flexibility. This relaxation can ease respiratory distress and contribute to improved respiratory function.

Anti-Inflammatory Effects: Cupping therapy has potential anti-inflammatory effects that can benefit individuals with respiratory disorders. Inflammation in the respiratory system can contribute to the symptoms and severity of respiratory conditions. Cupping therapy helps reduce inflammation by improving blood circulation, reducing oxidative stress, and modulating the immune response. By addressing inflammation, cupping therapy can help alleviate symptoms and promote overall respiratory well-being.

Complementary Therapy: Cupping therapy can be used as a complementary therapy alongside other treatments for respiratory disorders. It can enhance the effects of conventional treatments, such as medication, breathing exercises, and lifestyle modifications. By incorporating cupping therapy into a comprehensive treatment plan, individuals can optimize their respiratory management and improve their quality of life.

It is important to note that cupping therapy should be performed by trained professionals to ensure safe and effective treatment. The cups should be applied to clean and sanitized skin to minimize the risk of infection. Individuals with certain health conditions, such as bleeding disorders or skin infections, should consult their healthcare provider before undergoing cupping therapy.

Chapter Twenty-Two

Cupping Therapy for Digestive Disorders

Cupping therapy has gained recognition as a potential treatment for digestive disorders, offering a non-invasive and holistic approach to support digestive health. Digestive disorders encompass a range of conditions, including gastritis, irritable bowel syndrome (IBS), constipation, and indigestion. Cupping therapy provides potential benefits for symptom relief, improved digestion, and overall digestive well-being.

When it comes to digestive disorders, cupping therapy typically focuses on the abdominal area. The cups are applied to the abdomen to stimulate blood circulation, relax digestive muscles, and promote overall digestive function. Let's explore how cupping therapy can be beneficial for digestive disorders:

Pain Relief: Cupping therapy can provide pain relief for individuals with digestive disorders. The gentle suction created by the cups helps to relax the abdominal muscles and alleviate abdominal pain or cramping associated with conditions like gastritis or IBS. By improving blood circulation and promoting relaxation, cupping therapy can help reduce pain and discomfort in the digestive system.

Improved Digestion: Cupping therapy aids in improving digestion by promoting blood circulation and enhancing gastrointestinal function. The cups create a suction effect that stimulates the digestive organs, including the stomach and intestines, supporting the secretion of digestive enzymes and enhancing nutrient absorption. This can help individuals with digestive disorders experience improved digestion and reduced symptoms.

Reduction of Inflammation: Inflammation is a common factor in many digestive disorders and can contribute to symptoms such as abdominal pain, bloating, and diarrhea. Cupping therapy has shown potential in reducing inflammation through improved blood circulation, reduction of oxidative stress, and modulation of the immune response. By addressing inflammation, cupping therapy can help alleviate symptoms and promote overall digestive well-being.

Relaxation of Digestive Muscles: Cupping therapy helps to relax the muscles in the digestive system, aiding in the relief of digestive disorders. The gentle suction applied to the abdominal area stimulates blood circulation, induces a state of relaxation, and reduces muscle tension in the digestive organs. This relaxation can help alleviate spasms, cramping, and discomfort associated with digestive disorders.

Complementary Therapy: Cupping therapy can be used as a complementary therapy alongside other treatments for digestive disorders. It can enhance the effects of dietary modifications, medication, and lifestyle changes. By incorporating cupping therapy into a comprehensive treatment plan, individuals can optimize their digestive management and improve their quality of life.

It is important to note that cupping therapy should be performed by trained professionals to ensure safe and effective treatment. The cups should be applied to clean and sanitized skin to minimize the risk of infection. Individuals with certain health conditions, such as bleeding disorders or skin infections, should consult their healthcare provider before undergoing cupping therapy.

Chapter Twenty-Three

Cupping Therapy and Traditional Chinese Medicine

Cupping therapy is deeply rooted in Traditional Chinese Medicine (TCM) and has been practiced for centuries as a therapeutic modality. In TCM, cupping therapy is believed to promote the flow of Qi (vital energy) and blood, balance Yin and Yang energies, and restore health and well-being. This ancient healing practice offers a unique perspective on cupping therapy and its integration into holistic healthcare.

According to TCM principles, cupping therapy helps to remove stagnation and restore the free flow of Qi and blood in the body. Stagnation of Qi and blood is believed to be the underlying cause of various health conditions. The cups create suction on the skin, which helps to draw out stagnation, improve circulation, and restore balance.

Cupping therapy is often used to address imbalances in the body, such as pain, inflammation, and congestion. By applying cups to specific acupuncture points or meridian pathways, cupping therapy helps to stimulate the flow of Qi and blood along these channels, promoting balance and healing. The cups can be left in place or moved along the meridians to target specific areas of disharmony.

In TCM, cupping therapy is also used as a diagnostic tool. The appearance of the skin after cupping, including the coloration and markings, provides valuable information about the individual's health and the state of Qi and blood circulation. Practitioners can interpret these marks to gain insights into the underlying imbalances and tailor treatment accordingly.

Different techniques are used in cupping therapy within the context of TCM. The most common methods include stationary cupping, moving cupping, and flash cupping. Stationary cupping involves placing the cups on specific acupuncture points or areas of concern and leaving them in place for a certain duration. Moving cupping involves sliding the cups along the meridians, creating a massage-like effect. Flash cupping involves applying and removing the cups quickly to stimulate blood flow and energy movement.

Cupping therapy in TCM is often combined with other modalities, such as acupuncture, herbal medicine, and dietary recommendations, to provide a comprehensive treatment approach. These modalities work together to address the root causes of imbalances and support the body's innate healing capacity.

It is important to note that TCM-based cupping therapy should be performed by trained and qualified practitioners who have a deep understanding of the principles and techniques involved. This ensures safe and effective treatment and avoids potential complications.

While cupping therapy in TCM has been used for centuries, it is gaining recognition and popularity in the Western world as well. Modern research is exploring the mechanisms and benefits of cupping therapy, providing scientific evidence to support its efficacy. This integration of traditional wisdom with modern scientific understanding contributes to the broader acceptance and utilization of cupping therapy as a valuable healing modality.

Chapter Twenty-Four

The Meridian System

The meridian system is a fundamental concept in Traditional Chinese Medicine (TCM) and plays a significant role in cupping therapy. It is an intricate network of energy channels through which Qi (vital energy) flows, connecting different parts of the body. Understanding the meridian system helps to comprehend the principles behind cupping therapy and its effectiveness in promoting health and well-being.

In TCM, there are twelve primary meridians, each corresponding to a specific organ system or function in the body. These meridians are named after the organs they are associated with, such as the Lung, Large Intestine, Stomach, Spleen, Heart, Small Intestine, Bladder, Kidney, Pericardium, Triple Burner (San Jiao), Gallbladder, and Liver meridians. Additionally, there are eight extraordinary meridians that serve as reservoirs of Qi and help regulate the flow of energy throughout the body.

The meridians are believed to be pathways through which Qi flows, nourishing the organs, tissues, and cells. Qi is considered the vital force that sustains life and maintains health. When Qi flows smoothly and harmoniously along the meridians, the body is in a state of balance and well-being. However, if there is an imbalance or blockage in the flow of Qi, it can lead to physical and emotional disharmony, and eventually manifest as illness or pain.

Cupping therapy in TCM is often applied along the meridians to address specific imbalances or health concerns. The cups are placed on acupuncture points or moved along the meridians, creating a suction effect that stimulates Qi flow and promotes the restoration of balance. By targeting the meridians associated with specific organs or functions, cupping therapy aims to regulate Qi and support the body's natural healing processes.

The meridian system is not only a physical pathway but also has a profound connection to the mind and emotions. According to TCM, each meridian is associated with certain emotions and psychological aspects. For example, the Liver meridian is linked to anger and frustration, while the Lung meridian is associated with grief and sadness. By addressing imbalances in the meridian system, cupping therapy can help restore emotional equilibrium and promote overall well-being.

Cupping therapy can also be used diagnostically to assess the state of the meridians. The marks left by the cups after treatment, such as coloration or discoloration of the skin, provide valuable information about the underlying imbalances and the flow of Qi along the meridians. Practitioners can interpret these marks to gain insights into the individual's health condition and tailor the treatment accordingly.

It is important to note that cupping therapy and the meridian system are deeply rooted in TCM philosophy and should be practiced by qualified professionals who have a thorough understanding of the principles and techniques involved. They can provide personalized treatment based on the specific needs of the individual and ensure safe and effective application of cupping therapy along the meridians.

Chapter Twenty-Five

Cupping Therapy and Qi

Cupping therapy is closely linked to the concept of Qi (pronounced "chee") in Traditional Chinese Medicine (TCM). Qi is considered the vital energy that flows throughout the body, maintaining health and well-being. Understanding the relationship between cupping therapy and Qi is key to comprehending the underlying principles and therapeutic effects of this ancient healing practice.

In TCM, it is believed that Qi flows through a network of energy channels called meridians, nourishing the organs, tissues, and cells. When Qi is abundant and flowing smoothly, the body is in a state of balance and good health. However, if there is an imbalance or blockage in the flow of Qi, it can result in pain, illness, or emotional distress.

Cupping therapy is thought to affect the flow of Qi in the body. The cups create a suction effect on the skin, which stimulates blood circulation and Qi movement along the meridians. This helps to remove stagnation, invigorate Qi, and restore the flow of energy in the body. By promoting the free flow of Qi, cupping therapy aims to support the body's natural healing processes and restore balance.

The cups used in cupping therapy are often placed on specific acupuncture points or moved along the meridians to target areas of Qi stagnation or imbalance. This helps to activate the Qi flow and restore harmony in the affected areas. The cups can also be applied to areas of pain or discomfort, as pain is often seen as a manifestation of Qi stagnation.

The marks left by cupping therapy, commonly referred to as cupping marks, are considered significant in assessing the state of Qi in the body. These marks can range from light pink to dark red or even purple, depending on the individual's constitution and the level of Qi stagnation. The appearance and coloration of the cupping marks provide valuable information about the underlying imbalances and the flow of Qi. Practitioners can interpret these marks to tailor treatment and address specific Qi disharmonies.

Cupping therapy not only influences Qi on a physical level but also has an impact on the mental and emotional aspects of well-being. In TCM, emotions are seen as manifestations of Qi and are closely connected to the organs. By restoring the flow of Qi through cupping therapy, it is believed that emotional imbalances can also be addressed. For example, cupping therapy applied to the back can help release tension and stagnation in the Liver meridian, which is associated with emotions such as anger and frustration.

It is important to note that cupping therapy should be performed by trained professionals who have a deep understanding of the principles of TCM. They can assess the individual's condition, identify Qi imbalances, and provide personalized treatment based on the specific needs of the individual.

Chapter Twenty-Six

Cupping Therapy and Yin and Yang

Cupping therapy, rooted in Traditional Chinese Medicine (TCM), is closely connected to the concept of Yin and Yang. Yin and Yang represent opposing but complementary forces that exist in the universe and within the human body. Understanding the relationship between cupping therapy and Yin and Yang is essential to grasp the underlying principles and therapeutic effects of this ancient healing practice.

In TCM, Yin and Yang are fundamental concepts that describe the dualistic nature of all things. Yin represents qualities such as darkness, cold, rest, and inward energy, while Yang represents qualities such as light, warmth, activity, and outward energy. Health is believed to be a state of balance and harmony between Yin and Yang energies within the body.

Cupping therapy is used to restore the balance between Yin and Yang. By creating a suction effect on the skin, cupping therapy aims to regulate the flow of Qi (vital energy) and blood, which are considered manifestations of Yin and Yang. The cups are applied to specific acupuncture points or areas of concern to target imbalances and restore the harmony between Yin and Yang energies.

When there is an imbalance in Yin and Yang energies, health problems may arise. Cupping therapy is used to address these imbalances and restore equilibrium. For instance, if there is an excess of Yin energy manifesting as coldness or stagnation, cupping therapy can be used to invigorate Yang energy and promote warmth and movement. Conversely, if there is an excess of Yang energy causing symptoms such as inflammation or fever, cupping therapy can be applied to promote the cooling and calming Yin energy.

Cupping therapy can be applied in different ways to balance Yin and Yang energies. For example, moving cupping involves gliding the cups along the meridians to stimulate the flow of Qi and promote the balance of Yin and Yang. On the other hand, stationary cupping involves leaving the cups in place to tonify or disperse the energies depending on the individual's condition. These techniques can be used flexibly to address specific imbalances and restore the harmony of Yin and Yang energies.

The marks left by cupping therapy provide valuable information about the balance of Yin and Yang energies in the body. The coloration and appearance of the cupping marks, ranging from light pink to dark red or even purple, can indicate the presence of excess or deficiency in Yin or Yang. By observing and interpreting these marks, practitioners can adjust the treatment plan to restore the appropriate balance between Yin and Yang.

It is important to note that cupping therapy and the concept of Yin and Yang should be practiced by trained professionals who have a deep understanding of TCM principles. They can assess the individual's condition, identify imbalances, and provide personalized treatment based on the specific needs of the individual.

Chapter Twenty-Seven

Cupping Therapy and Western Medicine

Cupping therapy, a traditional healing practice originating from various cultures, has garnered attention and interest in Western medicine. While Western medicine primarily follows evidence-based practices, cupping therapy is often viewed as a complementary or alternative therapy. The integration of cupping therapy with Western medicine brings together different perspectives and approaches to enhance patient care and well-being.

In recent years, there has been growing research on cupping therapy, aiming to evaluate its effectiveness and mechanisms of action from a Western medical perspective. Studies have explored the physiological effects of cupping therapy, such as increased blood flow, lymphatic drainage, and tissue relaxation. Additionally, research has investigated its potential benefits in pain management, wound healing, and certain health conditions.

Cupping therapy is often used in conjunction with Western medicine to provide holistic care. It can be incorporated into treatment plans for various conditions, such as musculoskeletal disorders, sports injuries, and chronic pain. For example, in the field of sports medicine, cupping therapy is frequently used by athletes to support muscle recovery and alleviate pain.

One area where cupping therapy has gained recognition in Western medicine is pain management. The suction created by the cups stimulates sensory receptors, leading to pain modulation and increased local blood circulation. Cupping therapy has shown promise in relieving pain associated with conditions like back pain, neck pain, and migraines.

Moreover, cupping therapy has been explored as a potential treatment for certain dermatological conditions. In Western medicine, cupping therapy is sometimes used for managing conditions such as acne, eczema, and herpes zoster. The cups' suction effect can increase blood flow and improve the delivery of nutrients to the skin, promoting healing and reducing inflammation.

While cupping therapy is becoming more accepted in Western medicine, it is important to approach it with caution and adhere to best practices. Cupping therapy should be performed by trained professionals who understand proper techniques, hygiene, and safety precautions. Adverse effects such as skin irritation or bruising can occur if cupping therapy is administered incorrectly.

Collaboration between Western medicine practitioners and cupping therapy practitioners can provide comprehensive care for patients. By combining Western medical knowledge and diagnostic tools with the holistic approach of cupping therapy, healthcare providers can address both the physical and energetic aspects of a patient's well-being.

It is worth mentioning that cupping therapy is not meant to replace Western medical treatments, but rather to complement them. Patients are encouraged to consult with their healthcare providers and inform them of any complementary therapies they are considering. This allows for an open dialogue, ensuring the safe integration of cupping therapy into the overall treatment plan.

Chapter Twenty-Eight

Scientific Studies on Cupping Therapy

Scientific studies on cupping therapy have gained traction in recent years as researchers seek to evaluate its efficacy and understand its underlying mechanisms. While cupping therapy has been practiced for centuries, the scientific exploration aims to provide evidence-based support for its use and shed light on its potential benefits and applications.

One area of focus in scientific studies on cupping therapy is pain management. Several studies have shown promising results in reducing pain associated with various conditions. For example, a systematic review and meta-analysis published in the Journal of Traditional Chinese Medical Sciences found that cupping therapy was effective in relieving pain in individuals with chronic neck and shoulder pain. Another study published in the Journal of Pain Research demonstrated the positive effects of cupping therapy in reducing pain intensity and improving physical function in individuals with knee osteoarthritis.

Furthermore, scientific studies have examined the effects of cupping therapy on inflammation. In a study published in the Journal of Alternative and Complementary Medicine, researchers investigated the anti-inflammatory effects of cupping therapy in individuals with chronic low back pain. The results showed a significant reduction in inflammatory markers, indicating the potential of cupping therapy in managing inflammation.

Cupping therapy has also been explored in the context of skin conditions. A study published in the Journal of Cosmetic Dermatology examined the effects of cupping therapy on acne vulgaris. The findings demonstrated a significant reduction in acne lesions and improved skin appearance, supporting the use of cupping therapy as a complementary treatment for acne.

Moreover, scientific studies have delved into the physiological effects of cupping therapy. Research has shown that cupping therapy can increase local blood circulation, enhance lymphatic drainage, and improve tissue oxygenation. These effects contribute to the potential benefits of cupping therapy in wound healing, muscle recovery, and detoxification.

While scientific studies provide valuable insights into cupping therapy, it is important to acknowledge that more research is needed to establish a comprehensive understanding of its mechanisms and effectiveness. Many studies have limitations such as small sample sizes or lack of standardized protocols, which can impact the reliability of the findings. Nonetheless, the growing body of scientific research contributes to the knowledge base surrounding cupping therapy and provides a foundation for further investigation.

In addition to clinical studies, there have been efforts to explore the physiological and biochemical changes that occur during cupping therapy. Research utilizing technologies like ultrasound, magnetic resonance imaging (MRI), and biochemical analysis has provided insights into the mechanisms of cupping therapy. These studies have revealed changes in blood flow, tissue oxygenation, and the release of various substances, such as anti-inflammatory cytokines and endorphins, which may contribute to the therapeutic effects of cupping therapy.

It is worth noting that scientific studies on cupping therapy often emphasize the need for rigorous research methodologies and standardized protocols. This ensures that findings are reliable, reproducible, and applicable to a wider population. Researchers also stress the importance of conducting comparative studies and investigating the long-term effects of cupping therapy to further understand its potential benefits and limitations.

Chapter Twenty-Nine

Cupping Therapy and Myofascial Release

Cupping therapy and myofascial release are two therapeutic modalities that share common ground in their approach to addressing musculoskeletal conditions and promoting overall well-being. While cupping therapy has a long history rooted in traditional healing practices, myofascial release is a relatively newer technique developed in the field of manual therapy. Understanding the relationship between cupping therapy and myofascial release sheds light on their complementary nature and their potential synergistic effects.

Myofascial release focuses on the fascia, a connective tissue that surrounds and supports muscles, bones, and organs throughout the body. It aims to release restrictions or adhesions within the fascia, thereby restoring mobility, reducing pain, and improving overall function. The goal is to promote balance and optimal alignment of the musculoskeletal system.

Cupping therapy, on the other hand, utilizes suction to create negative pressure on the skin, facilitating increased blood flow, lymphatic drainage, and tissue relaxation. It is often applied to specific areas of the body to address pain, inflammation, and muscle tension. Cupping therapy helps to release adhesions, improve circulation, and enhance the flow of Qi (vital energy) and blood.

Cupping therapy can be seen as a form of myofascial release, as the suction created by the cups can help mobilize and release fascial restrictions. The negative pressure applied through cupping therapy creates a lifting effect on the underlying tissues, including the fascia. This can help to separate adhered tissues, improve tissue glide, and promote fascial hydration and flexibility.

When cupping therapy and myofascial release are combined, they can enhance the therapeutic effects on the fascia and surrounding tissues. Cupping therapy can be used as a preparatory technique before myofascial release to warm up the tissues, improve blood circulation, and increase tissue pliability. This can facilitate deeper and more effective myofascial release techniques, allowing for a more thorough release of fascial restrictions and tension.

Additionally, cupping therapy can be used after myofascial release to further promote tissue recovery and relaxation. The negative pressure applied through cupping can help to flush out metabolic waste products, increase nutrient delivery to the tissues, and reduce post-treatment soreness.

Furthermore, cupping therapy and myofascial release both have potential effects on the nervous system. Cupping therapy stimulates sensory receptors on the skin, leading to a neural response that can help modulate pain signals and promote relaxation. Myofascial release, through the release of fascial restrictions, can also have a positive impact on the nervous system, reducing pain sensitivity and restoring proper neuromuscular function.

It is important to note that cupping therapy and myofascial release should be performed by trained professionals who have a thorough understanding of the techniques and appropriate application. Each individual's condition should be assessed, and treatment should be tailored to their specific needs.

Chapter Thirty

Cupping Therapy and Sports Medicine

Cupping therapy has gained recognition and popularity within the field of sports medicine due to its potential benefits in supporting athletic performance, injury prevention, and recovery. Athletes from various sports disciplines have embraced cupping therapy as a valuable addition to their training and rehabilitation routines. The integration of cupping therapy and sports medicine offers a holistic approach to athletic care and performance optimization.

One of the primary benefits of cupping therapy in sports medicine is its ability to promote muscle recovery and alleviate muscle soreness. Intense physical activity can lead to muscle fatigue, microtrauma, and the accumulation of metabolic waste products. Cupping therapy, through the application of suction on the skin, helps to increase blood flow, stimulate lymphatic drainage, and promote the removal of metabolic waste. This aids in reducing post-exercise muscle soreness and promoting faster recovery between training sessions or competitions.

In addition to muscle recovery, cupping therapy can assist in injury prevention and rehabilitation. By improving blood circulation and oxygenation to the muscles and surrounding tissues, cupping therapy helps to enhance tissue healing and repair processes. Athletes often use cupping therapy as part of their injury prevention strategies, targeting areas prone to tightness, stiffness, or susceptibility to injury. The therapy helps to relieve muscle tension, increase flexibility, and improve overall musculoskeletal balance, thereby reducing the risk of injuries.

Cupping therapy is particularly beneficial for addressing common sports-related conditions such as strains, sprains, and tendinitis. The cups can be applied directly to the affected areas or along the relevant meridians to facilitate healing, reduce inflammation, and promote pain relief. Cupping therapy can also be used in conjunction with other sports medicine modalities such as stretching, strengthening exercises, and manual therapy techniques for a comprehensive and integrative approach to treatment and rehabilitation.

Athletes often turn to cupping therapy during the competitive season to enhance their performance and maintain optimal physical condition. By improving blood circulation and reducing muscle tension, cupping therapy can help athletes achieve better muscle function, range of motion, and overall performance. It is commonly utilized in sports that require repetitive movements, such as swimming, running, and cycling, to address muscular imbalances and optimize performance.

The psychological benefits of cupping therapy are also relevant in sports medicine. Athletes face intense physical and mental pressures, and cupping therapy can provide relaxation and stress reduction. The therapy's soothing effect on the nervous system helps athletes unwind, improve sleep quality, and manage stress and anxiety associated with performance expectations and recovery.

It is important to note that cupping therapy should be performed by trained professionals who have a solid understanding of sports medicine principles and techniques. They can assess athletes' specific needs, tailor treatment plans, and ensure safe and effective application of cupping therapy.

Chapter Thirty-One

Cupping Therapy Safety and Precautions

Cupping therapy is generally considered safe when performed by trained professionals who adhere to proper techniques and safety precautions. However, it is essential to be aware of certain safety considerations and guidelines to ensure a positive and risk-free cupping therapy experience.

One of the primary safety considerations in cupping therapy is the selection of appropriate cups. Cups used in therapy should be specifically designed for cupping and made of materials that are safe for skin contact, such as glass, silicone, or plastic. Cups should be in good condition, without any cracks or damage that may compromise their effectiveness or safety.

Hygiene is another crucial aspect of cupping therapy. Cups and other equipment used in the therapy should be properly cleaned and sterilized before each use to prevent the risk of infection. Additionally, practitioners should follow standard hygiene practices, such as washing their hands thoroughly and using disposable gloves when necessary, to maintain a clean and sanitary environment.

Proper application of cups is essential to ensure safety and minimize the risk of adverse effects. Cups should be placed on intact skin and should not be applied to areas with open wounds, cuts, or active infections. It is crucial to avoid cupping over sensitive areas, such as the eyes, genitals, or major blood vessels. Cupping therapy should be avoided in individuals with bleeding disorders or those who are taking anticoagulant medications, as it may increase the risk of bleeding or bruising.

During cupping therapy, it is important to monitor the duration and intensity of suction applied. Excessive suction or prolonged cupping time can lead to discomfort, bruising, or skin irritation. The cups should not be left in one place for an extended period to prevent the formation of excessive marks or skin discoloration. Additionally, the suction intensity should be adjusted based on the individual's comfort level and tolerance.

Individuals receiving cupping therapy should communicate any discomfort or pain during the treatment to the practitioner. It is essential to maintain open communication with the practitioner, informing them about any pre-existing medical conditions, allergies, or medications being taken. This helps the practitioner tailor the treatment plan and ensure that cupping therapy is suitable and safe for the individual.

Pregnant women should exercise caution when considering cupping therapy. While cupping therapy is generally considered safe during pregnancy, it is advisable to consult with a healthcare provider or an experienced cupping therapy practitioner to assess the appropriateness and potential risks associated with the therapy during pregnancy.

After cupping therapy, it is common to experience temporary marks or discoloration on the skin. These marks are typically harmless and fade within a few days to a couple of weeks. However, if there are any concerns or if the marks do not subside within a reasonable period, it is advisable to seek medical attention.

Chapter Thirty-Two

Potential Side Effects of Cupping Therapy

Cupping therapy, a traditional healing modality, is generally safe and well-tolerated when performed by trained professionals. However, like any therapeutic intervention, there are potential side effects that individuals should be aware of. Understanding these potential side effects can help individuals make informed decisions and ensure a safe cupping therapy experience.

One of the most common side effects of cupping therapy is temporary skin discoloration or marks. These marks are caused by the suction applied to the skin and typically appear as circular or oval-shaped bruises. The discoloration can range in color from light pink to dark purple, depending on the individual's skin tone and the intensity of the suction. These marks usually fade within a few days to a couple of weeks, but in some cases, they may persist for longer.

Another possible side effect of cupping therapy is skin irritation or discomfort. The cups can create a pulling sensation on the skin, which may cause temporary discomfort or tenderness. In rare cases, cupping therapy may result in mild skin irritation, such as redness or itching. These effects are usually temporary and subside on their own.

In certain situations, cupping therapy may lead to more significant side effects. Excessive suction or prolonged cupping time can result in more pronounced bruising, skin damage, or even blistering. To prevent these complications, it is important for practitioners to use appropriate suction intensity and carefully monitor the treatment duration.

Individuals with certain health conditions or sensitivities may be more prone to experiencing side effects. For instance, individuals with sensitive skin, fragile blood vessels, or bleeding disorders may have a higher risk of developing bruises or skin irritation. It is crucial for individuals with such conditions to communicate their medical history to the cupping therapy practitioner, who can then adjust the treatment plan accordingly.

Pain during cupping therapy is generally mild and temporary. However, if an individual experiences severe pain during or after the treatment, it could indicate that the suction intensity was too strong or that the cups were left in place for an extended period. It is important to communicate any discomfort or pain to the practitioner during the treatment session so that adjustments can be made to ensure a more comfortable experience.

In rare cases, cupping therapy may cause dizziness or lightheadedness, particularly when performed on certain areas of the body or with excessive suction. This may be due to the local vasodilation caused by the therapy. If an individual feels lightheaded or dizzy during or after cupping therapy, it is important to rest and allow the symptoms to subside.

Pregnant women should exercise caution when considering cupping therapy, particularly on the abdomen or lower back. While there is limited research on the effects of cupping therapy during pregnancy, it is advisable for pregnant women to consult with their healthcare provider before undergoing the treatment.

It is important to note that severe or persistent side effects of cupping therapy are rare. However, if an individual experiences any concerning or unusual reactions following cupping therapy, it is advisable to seek medical attention.

Chapter Thirty-Three

Contraindications for Cupping Therapy

Cupping therapy is generally safe and well-tolerated, but there are certain situations in which it is contraindicated. Contraindications refer to specific conditions or circumstances in which the use of cupping therapy may be inappropriate or potentially harmful. It is important for individuals and practitioners to be aware of these contraindications to ensure the safe and effective application of cupping therapy.

One of the primary contraindications for cupping therapy is the presence of skin conditions or lesions in the treatment area. Open wounds, cuts, burns, or active skin infections are contraindications for cupping therapy. Applying cups to damaged or compromised skin can increase the risk of infection, delay wound healing, or exacerbate the existing condition. It is crucial to allow the skin to heal fully before considering cupping therapy in the affected area.

Individuals with a bleeding disorder or those taking anticoagulant medications should avoid cupping therapy or exercise caution. Cupping therapy can increase local blood circulation and may cause minor bleeding or bruising. Individuals with a bleeding disorder or those taking blood-thinning medications may be at a higher risk of excessive bleeding or bruising. It is important to consult with a healthcare provider before considering cupping therapy in such cases.

Cupping therapy should be avoided in areas of the body where there are major blood vessels or delicate structures. The cups should not be applied directly over large blood vessels, organs, the eyes, or genitals. Additionally, caution should be exercised in areas with bony prominences or thin skin, as they are more susceptible to bruising or discomfort during cupping therapy.

Individuals with a history of cancer or currently undergoing cancer treatment should consult with their healthcare provider before considering cupping therapy. While cupping therapy is generally well-tolerated, it is important to consider the potential effects on cancer-related treatments or conditions. The cups' suction may stimulate blood flow, and in some cases, this may not be desirable during cancer treatment.

Pregnant women should approach cupping therapy with caution. While there is limited research on the effects of cupping therapy during pregnancy, it is advisable for pregnant women to consult with their healthcare provider before undergoing the treatment. Special considerations and precautions may be necessary to ensure the safety of both the mother and the baby.

Individuals with certain systemic conditions or chronic diseases should also exercise caution when considering cupping therapy. Conditions such as hemophilia, deep vein thrombosis, severe edema, severe heart or kidney disease, and uncontrolled hypertension may be contraindications or require modified cupping techniques. It is important to consult with a healthcare provider to determine the appropriateness of cupping therapy in these cases.

Furthermore, individuals with a history of skin sensitivity or allergic reactions should inform the cupping therapy practitioner before the treatment. This allows the practitioner to select cups and techniques that are suitable for the individual's skin condition and minimize the risk of adverse reactions.

Chapter Thirty-Four

Cupping Therapy and Pregnancy

Cupping therapy is a traditional healing modality that has gained popularity in recent years. However, when it comes to cupping therapy during pregnancy, caution and informed decision-making are essential. Pregnancy is a unique physiological state, and certain considerations must be taken into account to ensure the safety and well-being of both the mother and the baby.

One of the primary concerns with cupping therapy during pregnancy is the potential impact on the developing fetus. While cupping therapy is generally considered safe, there is limited research specifically focusing on its effects during pregnancy. Therefore, it is advisable for pregnant women to consult with their healthcare provider before considering cupping therapy.

The location and intensity of cupping therapy during pregnancy are important factors to consider. Cupping therapy should be avoided on the abdomen or lower back, especially during the first trimester. These areas are in close proximity to the developing fetus and the uterus, and the effects of cupping therapy on these regions are not well-understood. However, cupping therapy on other areas of the body, such as the upper back or shoulders, may be considered with caution and proper positioning.

Another consideration is the suction intensity used during cupping therapy. Gentle and moderate suction is typically recommended during pregnancy to minimize any potential risks or discomfort. High-intensity suction should be avoided, as it may lead to increased blood flow or possible complications.

Individuals who have experienced complications during previous pregnancies or those with a high-risk pregnancy should exercise greater caution when considering cupping therapy. In these cases, it is advisable to consult with a healthcare provider who can provide personalized advice based on the individual's specific circumstances.

During pregnancy, hormonal changes can lead to increased skin sensitivity. It is important for pregnant women to communicate any changes or concerns regarding their skin to the cupping therapy practitioner. This allows the practitioner to select cups and techniques that are suitable for the individual's skin condition and minimize the risk of adverse reactions or skin irritation.

Additionally, pregnant women should be aware of their comfort levels during cupping therapy. Pregnancy can cause changes in posture, weight distribution, and discomfort in certain positions. It is crucial to communicate any discomfort or concerns to the cupping therapy practitioner during the session. The practitioner can then adjust the positioning and techniques to ensure a comfortable experience for the pregnant individual.

Pregnant women considering cupping therapy should also be mindful of their overall prenatal care and consult with their healthcare provider. Cupping therapy should be seen as a complementary modality rather than a substitute for routine prenatal care. It is important to continue regular prenatal check-ups and follow the guidance of the healthcare provider throughout the pregnancy journey.

Chapter Thirty-Five

Cupping Therapy Equipment

Cupping therapy is a traditional healing modality that utilizes specialized equipment to create suction on the skin. The equipment used in cupping therapy plays a crucial role in ensuring the effectiveness and safety of the treatment. Let's explore the various types of cupping therapy equipment commonly used in practice.

Cups: Cups are the primary equipment used in cupping therapy. They are available in different materials such as glass, silicone, plastic, or bamboo. Glass cups are most commonly used in traditional cupping therapy, while silicone and plastic cups are popular in modern practice due to their flexibility and ease of use. Bamboo cups are less common but can be used in certain traditional cupping techniques. Cups come in various sizes, allowing practitioners to select the appropriate size for different treatment areas.

Suction Devices: Suction devices are used to create the negative pressure required for cupping therapy. Traditional methods involve using handheld suction pumps, which are manually operated to create suction in the cups. Modern cupping therapy often utilizes mechanical suction devices, such as electric pumps or suction machines, which allow for more precise control over the suction intensity.

Fire: In traditional fire cupping, fire is briefly introduced inside the cup to create a vacuum. The fire consumes the oxygen inside the cup, creating a negative pressure when the cup is placed on the skin. This method requires the use of specialized fire-resistant cups. Fire cupping should only be performed by trained professionals who follow strict safety protocols to prevent accidents or burns.

Alcohol or Cotton Balls: Alcohol or cotton balls soaked in alcohol are used in fire cupping to ignite the fire inside the cup. The alcohol-soaked cotton ball is lit and briefly placed inside the cup before being removed and quickly placed on the skin. This method requires caution and expertise to ensure the safety of both the practitioner and the patient.

Lubricants: Lubricants such as massage oil or lotion are often used in cupping therapy to help the cups glide smoothly over the skin. Applying a small amount of lubricant to the treatment area minimizes friction, allowing for easier cup placement and movement. It also enhances the comfort of the patient during the therapy.

Cleaning and Sterilization Supplies: Proper cleaning and sterilization of cupping equipment are essential to maintain hygiene and prevent the risk of infection. Healthcare professionals follow specific protocols for cleaning and sterilizing cups between treatments. Common cleaning supplies include soap, water, and disinfectants. Sterilization may involve autoclaving or using specialized sterilization equipment.

Storage and Carrying Cases: Cupping therapy equipment can be stored and transported in specialized cases designed to protect the cups and other accessories. These cases help keep the equipment organized, easily accessible, and protected from damage during storage or travel.

It is important for cupping therapy practitioners to ensure the quality and safety of their equipment. Cups should be free from cracks or damage that could compromise their effectiveness or safety. Suction devices should be well-maintained and calibrated to provide consistent suction. Additionally, proper cleaning and sterilization of equipment between treatments are crucial to prevent the risk of cross-contamination and infection.

Chapter Thirty-Six

Cups

Cups are the central equipment used in cupping therapy, and they play a vital role in the effectiveness and success of the treatment. These specialized vessels create suction on the skin, promoting various therapeutic effects. Let's explore the different types of cups used in cupping therapy and their characteristics.

Glass Cups: Glass cups are the most commonly used cups in traditional cupping therapy. They are made of thick, durable glass and come in various sizes. Glass cups have a smooth surface and provide good visibility, allowing practitioners to monitor the skin's response during the therapy. They are often used in stationary cupping or in techniques where fire is used to create suction.

Silicone Cups: Silicone cups have gained popularity in modern cupping therapy due to their flexibility, ease of use, and safety. These cups are made of medical-grade silicone, which is soft, pliable, and hypoallergenic. Silicone cups are transparent, allowing practitioners to observe the skin during the treatment. They also come in different sizes and can be used in both stationary and dynamic cupping techniques.

Plastic Cups: Plastic cups are another option in cupping therapy. They are made of durable plastic material and are lightweight and portable. Plastic cups are available in various sizes and shapes, including both traditional round cups and newer designs with built-in suction mechanisms. Plastic cups are suitable for both stationary and dynamic cupping techniques.

Bamboo Cups: Bamboo cups are less common but still used in some traditional cupping practices. These cups are handmade from bamboo and have a unique shape and design. They are generally larger in size and may be used for both stationary and sliding cupping techniques. Bamboo cups provide a more rustic and traditional feel to the cupping therapy experience.

Each type of cup has its own advantages and considerations. Glass cups provide excellent visibility, while silicone and plastic cups offer flexibility and ease of use. Bamboo cups offer a traditional touch and may appeal to those seeking an authentic cupping therapy experience.

Cupping therapy cups come in different sizes to accommodate various body areas and treatment objectives. Smaller cups are commonly used for facial cupping or in delicate areas, while larger cups are suitable for broader body areas such as the back or thighs. The cups' sizes can be selected based on the practitioner's expertise and the patient's comfort level.

In addition to the material and size, cups can also have different designs and features. Some cups have a valve mechanism that allows for easy suction control, while others require manual suction using handheld pumps or fire. Cupping sets may include cups with different shapes, such as rounded cups for stationary cupping and elongated cups for sliding cupping.

Regardless of the cup type, it is important for cupping therapy practitioners to ensure the cups are in good condition, free from cracks or damage that could compromise their effectiveness or safety. Proper cleaning and sterilization of the cups between treatments are essential to maintain hygiene and prevent the risk of infection.

Chapter Thirty-Seven

Cupping Sets

Cupping sets are specialized kits that contain multiple cups of various sizes and sometimes additional accessories used in cupping therapy. These sets provide practitioners with a range of cup sizes and options for different body areas and treatment techniques. Let's delve into the features and benefits of cupping sets in the context of cupping therapy.

Variety of Cup Sizes: Cupping sets typically include cups of different sizes, ranging from small to large. This variety allows practitioners to adapt the cup size to the specific treatment area and individual needs of the patient. Smaller cups are suitable for delicate areas such as the face or neck, while larger cups are better suited for larger body areas like the back or thighs. The availability of multiple cup sizes in a set enhances the versatility and effectiveness of cupping therapy.

Stationary and Sliding Cupping: Cupping sets often include both rounded cups for stationary cupping and elongated cups for sliding cupping techniques. Stationary cupping involves placing the cups on specific acupoints or areas of tension and leaving them in place for a designated period. Sliding cupping involves applying lubrication to the skin and using the cups to glide smoothly over the treatment area. The inclusion of cups for both techniques allows practitioners to perform a wide range of cupping methods based on the patient's needs.

Convenient Storage and Organization: Cupping sets typically come in a convenient storage case or bag, allowing practitioners to keep their cups organized and easily accessible. The storage case helps protect the cups from damage and allows for easy transportation between treatment locations. With proper organization, practitioners can quickly find the right cup size and set up their cupping therapy sessions efficiently.

Combination of Cup Materials: Cupping sets may include cups made from different materials such as glass, silicone, plastic, or bamboo. This combination of cup materials provides practitioners with options to cater to their own preferences or the patient's specific needs. For example, glass cups may be preferred for traditional cupping techniques, while silicone or plastic cups offer flexibility and ease of use. Bamboo cups may be chosen for those seeking a more traditional cupping experience.

Accessibility for Self-Treatment: Cupping sets also offer the benefit of accessibility for self-treatment. With a cupping set, individuals can perform cupping therapy on themselves in the comfort of their own homes. This allows for more frequent and convenient treatments without the need to visit a practitioner. However, it is important for individuals to educate themselves on proper cupping techniques and safety precautions before attempting self-treatment.

Cost-Effectiveness: Cupping sets can be a cost-effective option for practitioners who frequently use cupping therapy in their practice. Instead of purchasing individual cups separately, a cupping set provides a range of cup sizes and styles at a bundled price. This can be more economical in the long run, especially for practitioners who offer cupping therapy as a regular treatment option.

It is important to note that cupping sets should be selected based on their quality and adherence to safety standards. Cups should be free from cracks or defects that could compromise their effectiveness or safety. Practitioners should also follow proper cleaning and sterilization protocols to maintain hygiene and prevent the risk of infection.

Chapter Thirty-Eight

Cupping Therapy Accessories

Cupping therapy accessories are additional tools and supplies used in conjunction with cups to enhance the cupping therapy experience and provide additional therapeutic benefits. These accessories complement the use of cups and contribute to the overall effectiveness of the treatment. Let's explore some common cupping therapy accessories and their roles in the practice.

Cupping Oil or Lubricant: Cupping oil or lubricant is used to facilitate the movement of cups on the skin during sliding cupping techniques. Applying a small amount of cupping oil or lubricant to the treatment area reduces friction, allowing the cups to glide smoothly over the skin. This enhances the comfort of the patient and allows for better control and manipulation of the cups during the treatment.

Cupping Magnets: Cupping magnets are small magnets that can be attached to the cups to provide additional therapeutic effects. These magnets are often used in magnetic cupping, where the magnets create a magnetic field that interacts with the body's energy channels or acupoints. Magnetic cupping is believed to promote balance and harmony in the body, aiding in the restoration of health.

Cupping Massage Tools: Cupping massage tools, such as silicone or plastic suction cups with built-in rollers or knobs, combine the benefits of cupping therapy with massage techniques. These tools allow practitioners to simultaneously apply suction and perform massage movements over the treatment area. Cupping massage tools can help relieve muscle tension, improve blood circulation, and enhance the relaxation and therapeutic effects of the treatment.

Gua Sha Tools: Gua sha tools are smooth-edged instruments typically made of jade, horn, or other materials. They are used in conjunction with cupping therapy to enhance the therapeutic benefits. After cupping treatment, the skin may be gently scraped using the gua sha tool in a specific manner. This scraping action helps stimulate blood circulation, release muscle tension, and promote lymphatic drainage, further enhancing the overall effectiveness of cupping therapy.

Cupping Pumps: Cupping pumps are handheld devices used to create suction in the cups. They provide a controlled and consistent method of generating suction, eliminating the need for manual suction or fire in traditional cupping. Cupping pumps allow practitioners to adjust the suction intensity to suit individual needs and treatment goals. They are especially useful for practitioners who perform cupping therapy frequently and require a reliable and efficient way to create suction.

Cleaning and Sterilization Supplies: Proper cleaning and sterilization of cupping accessories are crucial to maintain hygiene and prevent the risk of infection. Accessories such as cups, gua sha tools, or cupping massage tools should be cleaned and sterilized following appropriate protocols between each use. Cleaning supplies include soap, water, and disinfectants, while sterilization may involve autoclaving or using specialized sterilization equipment.

Educational Materials: Educational materials such as books, DVDs, or online resources play a significant role in cupping therapy practice. These materials provide practitioners with knowledge on cupping techniques, indications, contraindications, and best practices. They serve as valuable resources for practitioners to enhance their skills and expand their understanding of cupping therapy.

It is important to note that cupping therapy accessories should be of high quality and meet safety standards. Cups, cupping massage tools, or gua sha tools should be free from defects or damage that could compromise their effectiveness or safety. Additionally, proper cleaning and sterilization protocols should be followed to ensure the accessories' cleanliness and prevent the risk of cross-contamination.

Chapter Thirty-Nine

Cupping Therapy Procedure

Cupping therapy is a traditional healing modality that involves creating suction on the skin using specialized cups. The procedure of cupping therapy follows a specific sequence to ensure its effectiveness and safety. Let's explore the general steps involved in a cupping therapy session.

Consultation and Assessment: Before starting the cupping therapy procedure, a practitioner typically conducts a consultation and assessment with the patient. This allows the practitioner to gather information about the patient's medical history, current health condition, and specific concerns. The practitioner may also perform a physical examination or palpation to identify areas of tension or stagnation that may benefit from cupping therapy.

Cup Selection: Based on the assessment and treatment goals, the practitioner selects the appropriate cups for the session. Cups come in various sizes, and the selection depends on the treatment area and the desired therapeutic effects. Smaller cups may be used for targeted areas or delicate regions, while larger cups are suitable for broader body areas.

Preparation of the Treatment Area: The treatment area is prepared by cleaning and disinfecting the skin to maintain hygiene. If necessary, cupping oil or lubricant may be applied to the skin to facilitate the movement of the cups during the therapy.

Cup Placement: The cups are placed on the skin by creating suction. There are different methods to achieve this suction, depending on the cupping technique used. Traditional cupping methods involve the use of fire or manual suction pumps to create a vacuum inside the cups. Modern cupping methods often utilize mechanical suction devices or cups with built-in suction mechanisms. The cups are placed firmly on the skin, and the suction creates a pulling sensation.

Cup Duration: The cups are left in place for a designated period, typically ranging from a few minutes to around 20 minutes. The duration may vary depending on factors such as the patient's tolerance, treatment goals, and the cupping technique used. During this time, the cups may remain stationary or may be gently moved or manipulated to enhance the therapeutic effects.

Cup Removal: After the desired duration, the cups are carefully removed from the skin. This is done by breaking the seal created by the suction, which can be achieved by pressing on the skin near the cup's edge or using a release valve mechanism, depending on the cupping equipment used.

Post-Cupping Care: After cup removal, the practitioner may provide post-treatment care instructions to the patient. This may include recommendations for hydration, rest, or avoiding excessive heat or cold immediately after the session. It is common to observe temporary marks on the skin from the cupping therapy, which are usually harmless and fade within a few days.

It is important to note that cupping therapy should be performed by trained professionals who have a thorough understanding of the technique and its applications. They should adhere to proper hygiene and safety practices, including the use of clean cups and appropriate disinfection protocols between each session.

The frequency and number of cupping therapy sessions may vary depending on the individual's condition and response to treatment. Some individuals may require multiple sessions spread over a specific timeframe for optimal results, while others may benefit from occasional or maintenance sessions.

Chapter Forty

Preparing for Cupping Therapy

Preparing for cupping therapy is an important step to ensure a safe and effective treatment session. Proper preparation helps both the practitioner and the patient make the most out of the therapy. Let's explore some key aspects of preparing for cupping therapy.

Consultation and Assessment: Before undergoing cupping therapy, it is advisable to schedule a consultation with a qualified cupping therapy practitioner. During this consultation, the practitioner will assess your medical history, current health condition, and any specific concerns you may have. This assessment helps determine if cupping therapy is suitable for you and allows the practitioner to tailor the treatment to your individual needs.

Hydration: Staying well-hydrated is important before cupping therapy. Adequate hydration helps improve blood circulation and prepares the body for the therapy. It is recommended to drink plenty of water in the days leading up to your session and continue to hydrate on the day of the treatment.

Skin Care: Taking care of your skin before cupping therapy is crucial for both comfort and hygiene. Ensure that the treatment area is clean and free from lotions, oils, or any substances that may interfere with the cupping process. If necessary, the practitioner may provide specific instructions regarding skin preparation before the session.

Clothing Choice: Choosing appropriate clothing for your cupping therapy session is essential for comfort and ease of access to the treatment areas. Loose-fitting and comfortable clothing is recommended, as it allows easy access to the areas where the cups will be applied. It is also important to consider modesty and choose clothing that makes you feel at ease during the session.

Discuss Expectations and Concerns: Before the session, take the opportunity to discuss your expectations and any concerns you may have with the practitioner. Open communication helps ensure that both you and the practitioner are on the same page and allows for a more personalized treatment approach. You can discuss your goals, any specific areas of concern, and ask any questions you may have about the therapy.

Mental and Emotional Preparation: Cupping therapy is not only a physical treatment but also an opportunity for relaxation and emotional well-being. Prior to your session, take a few moments to relax, clear your mind, and mentally prepare for the therapy. Practicing deep breathing or meditation techniques can help you achieve a state of relaxation and enhance the overall therapeutic benefits of the session.

Post-Treatment Plan: It is important to have a post-treatment plan in place to maximize the benefits of cupping therapy. The practitioner may provide recommendations for post-treatment care, which may include avoiding strenuous activities, applying specific ointments or oils, or engaging in self-care practices such as stretching or relaxation exercises. Following the post-treatment plan can help maintain the effects of cupping therapy and support your overall well-being.

It is crucial to consult a qualified cupping therapy practitioner who has the necessary training and experience to perform the therapy safely and effectively. They can provide personalized guidance on preparing for your cupping therapy session based on your specific needs and health condition.

Chapter Forty-One

Cupping Therapy Session

A cupping therapy session involves a series of steps that are designed to provide a safe and effective treatment experience. From the moment you arrive at the practitioner's office to the end of the session, each step is carefully executed to ensure optimal therapeutic benefits. Let's explore the various components of a cupping therapy session.

Greeting and Preparation: When you arrive for your cupping therapy session, the practitioner will greet you and guide you to the treatment room. They will take a few moments to understand any specific concerns you may have and answer any questions you may ask. This initial interaction helps create a comfortable and supportive environment for the session.

Assessment and Discussion: Before proceeding with the cupping therapy, the practitioner will conduct a brief assessment to determine the treatment areas and cupping techniques that are most suitable for you. They may ask about your medical history, current health condition, and any specific goals you have for the therapy. This discussion allows the practitioner to tailor the session to your individual needs.

Preparation of the Treatment Area: Once the assessment is complete, the practitioner will prepare the treatment area. This typically involves cleaning and disinfecting the skin to maintain hygiene. If necessary, cupping oil or lubricant may be applied to the skin to ensure smooth movement of the cups during the session.

Cup Placement: The practitioner will then begin the cupping therapy by placing the cups on the treatment areas. Depending on the cupping technique being used, the cups may be applied directly to the skin or moved in a sliding motion. The cups create suction, which promotes blood circulation, releases muscle tension, and stimulates the body's natural healing response.

Suction Control and Comfort: Throughout the session, the practitioner will monitor the suction intensity and ensure your comfort. If at any point the suction feels too strong or uncomfortable, the practitioner can adjust the suction or move the cups to alleviate any discomfort. Open communication between you and the practitioner is encouraged during the session to ensure a comfortable experience.

Duration of Cupping: The cups are typically left in place for a designated period, which can range from a few minutes to around 20 minutes. The duration depends on various factors, including the cupping technique, your comfort level, and the treatment goals. During this time, you may feel sensations such as a pulling or warmth around the cups, which is a normal part of the cupping therapy experience.

Cup Removal and Post-Cupping Care: Once the designated time has elapsed, the practitioner will carefully remove the cups from your skin. They will release the suction by breaking the seal created by the cups. After cup removal, the practitioner may provide post-cupping care instructions. This may include recommendations for hydration, rest, or avoiding activities that may strain the treated areas. The practitioner may also address any post-treatment questions or concerns you may have.

Follow-up and Treatment Plan: Depending on your specific needs, the practitioner may recommend a treatment plan that includes multiple cupping therapy sessions. They may discuss the frequency and number of sessions required to achieve the desired therapeutic outcomes. Follow-up appointments allow the practitioner to track your progress and adjust the treatment plan as needed.

Throughout the session, the practitioner will maintain a professional and supportive atmosphere, ensuring your comfort and well-being. They will prioritize your safety by using clean and sterilized cups and following hygiene protocols. It is important to communicate any sensations or discomfort you experience during the session to the practitioner for appropriate adjustments.

Chapter Forty-Two

Aftercare for Cupping Therapy

Aftercare for cupping therapy is an important aspect of the treatment process that helps optimize the therapeutic benefits and promote overall well-being. It involves taking certain precautions and engaging in self-care practices to support the body's healing process after a cupping therapy session. Let's explore some essential aftercare steps to follow.

Hydration: Drinking an adequate amount of water is crucial after cupping therapy. Hydration helps flush out toxins released during the treatment and supports the body's natural detoxification process. Aim to drink plenty of water in the hours and days following the session to stay hydrated and promote optimal healing.

Rest and Relaxation: After cupping therapy, it is advisable to allow yourself some time for rest and relaxation. The therapy stimulates the body's healing response and can leave you feeling relaxed and rejuvenated. Take the opportunity to engage in activities that promote rest and relaxation, such as taking a warm bath, practicing deep breathing exercises, or enjoying a gentle walk in nature.

Avoiding Excessive Heat or Cold: It is recommended to avoid exposure to excessive heat or cold immediately after cupping therapy. This includes activities such as hot showers, saunas, or intense physical exercise. Extreme temperatures can affect the body's response to the therapy and may disrupt the healing process. Opt for moderate temperature environments and activities until your body has fully adjusted.

Gentle Stretching and Movement: Engaging in gentle stretching and movement exercises can help maintain the benefits of cupping therapy. These activities promote flexibility, improve blood circulation, and prevent muscle stiffness. However, avoid vigorous or strenuous exercise for at least 24 to 48 hours after the session to allow your body to recover.

Skin Care: Proper skin care after cupping therapy is essential to ensure the well-being of your skin. Avoid applying any creams, lotions, or oils to the cupping marks or treated areas immediately after the session. Allow the skin to breathe and heal naturally. Over time, the cupping marks will fade on their own, but it is important to protect the skin from excessive sun exposure and apply a moisturizer to keep it hydrated.

Communication with the Practitioner: If you have any concerns or questions after the cupping therapy session, do not hesitate to reach out to your practitioner. They can provide guidance and answer any queries you may have regarding post-treatment care. It is important to follow their instructions and recommendations to ensure optimal healing and address any potential issues.

Follow-Up Sessions: Depending on your specific needs and treatment goals, your practitioner may recommend follow-up cupping therapy sessions. These sessions are designed to build upon the initial treatment and provide continued support for your well-being. Adhering to the recommended schedule and attending follow-up sessions can help maintain the benefits of cupping therapy and address any persistent concerns.

Remember that each individual's response to cupping therapy may vary, and the aftercare instructions may differ based on your unique circumstances. It is essential to consult with your practitioner for personalized aftercare guidance tailored to your specific needs.

Chapter Forty-Three

Cupping Therapy and Self-Care

Cupping therapy is not only a treatment modality but also a form of self-care that can be incorporated into your wellness routine. By combining cupping therapy with self-care practices, you can enhance the therapeutic benefits and promote your overall well-being. Let's explore how cupping therapy can be integrated into a self-care regimen.

Mindful Relaxation: Cupping therapy provides an opportunity for mindful relaxation. During the session, you can embrace a state of calmness and mindfulness, allowing yourself to fully experience the sensations and benefits of the therapy. By focusing on your breath and being present in the moment, cupping therapy becomes a meditative practice that promotes relaxation and stress reduction.

Self-Reflection and Intention Setting: Prior to your cupping therapy session, take a few moments for self-reflection and intention setting. Set clear intentions for the session, whether it's to release tension, improve energy flow, or promote physical and emotional healing. By setting intentions, you cultivate a sense of purpose and direction, enhancing the therapeutic effects of the therapy.

Incorporating Essential Oils: Essential oils can be a valuable addition to your cupping therapy self-care routine. You can use essential oils known for their relaxing or invigorating properties, such as lavender, chamomile, or peppermint. Apply a few drops of the selected oil to the skin before the cupping therapy session to enhance the sensory experience and promote a sense of well-being.

Self-Massage: After cupping therapy, incorporate self-massage into your routine to extend the benefits of the treatment. Gently massage the areas where the cups were applied to further stimulate blood circulation, release muscle tension, and promote lymphatic drainage. You can use your hands or incorporate massage tools to enhance the self-massage experience.

Stretching and Movement: Engaging in gentle stretching and movement exercises following cupping therapy can be an effective form of self-care. Stretching helps maintain flexibility, prevents muscle stiffness, and promotes overall physical well-being. Incorporate stretching into your post-cupping routine to maximize the therapeutic effects and support your body's healing process.

Hydration and Nutrition: Hydration and proper nutrition are essential aspects of self-care that can complement cupping therapy. Drink plenty of water after the session to support detoxification and hydration. Additionally, focus on consuming a balanced diet rich in nutrients to support your body's healing and overall well-being.

Self-Reflection and Journaling: Take some time after your cupping therapy session for self-reflection and journaling. Reflect on your experience, the sensations you felt during the session, and any insights or emotions that arose. Journaling can be a powerful tool for self-discovery, stress management, and personal growth.

Regular Self-Care Routine: Cupping therapy can be integrated into a regular self-care routine. Consider incorporating cupping therapy sessions on a regular basis to support your overall well-being. Schedule regular appointments to create a consistent self-care practice that nurtures your physical, mental, and emotional health.

Remember that self-care is a personal journey, and it's important to listen to your body and honor your needs. If you have any specific health concerns or questions, consult with a qualified cupping therapy practitioner to ensure that cupping therapy is appropriate for you and complements your self-care routine.

Chapter Forty-Four

Self-Care Cupping Techniques

Self-care cupping techniques offer individuals the opportunity to harness the therapeutic benefits of cupping therapy in the comfort of their own homes. By learning and applying these techniques, you can incorporate cupping therapy into your self-care routine and promote your overall well-being. Let's explore some self-care cupping techniques that you can easily practice.

Facial Cupping: Facial cupping is a popular self-care technique that promotes healthy skin and relaxation. To perform facial cupping, start by applying a facial oil or serum to clean, dry skin. Then, using small facial cups, create a gentle suction on different areas of your face, such as the forehead, cheeks, and jawline. Glide the cups in upward and outward motions, following the natural contours of your face. Facial cupping can help improve blood circulation, reduce puffiness, and enhance the appearance of the skin.

Back Cupping: Back cupping is an effective self-care technique for releasing tension and promoting relaxation in the back muscles. You can use silicone cups or suction cups designed for self-use. Apply a small amount of oil or lotion to the area you want to treat, then place the cup on the skin and create suction. Gently glide the cup along your back, focusing on areas of tension or discomfort. Back cupping can help alleviate muscle tightness, improve circulation, and promote a sense of relaxation.

Cellulite Cupping: Cellulite cupping is a technique that targets areas affected by cellulite, such as the thighs, buttocks, and abdomen. Apply a cellulite massage oil or lotion to the area, then use silicone cups or cellulite-specific cups to create suction. Glide the cups over the cellulite-affected areas using a combination of long strokes and circular motions. This technique can help stimulate blood flow, reduce the appearance of cellulite, and improve the tone and texture of the skin.

Reflexology Cupping: Reflexology cupping combines the principles of reflexology with cupping therapy. It involves applying suction cups to specific reflex points on the feet, hands, or ears. Apply a small amount of oil or lotion to the area, then place the cup on the reflex point and create suction. Leave the cup in place for a few minutes or gently glide it over the reflex points. Reflexology cupping can help promote relaxation, stimulate the corresponding organs or systems, and support overall balance and well-being.

Energy Balancing Cupping: Energy balancing cupping involves using cups to stimulate energy meridians and promote a sense of balance and harmony within the body. Apply a small amount of oil to the area, then place the cup on a specific energy point, such as along the meridian pathways or acupuncture points. Create suction and gently glide or hold the cups in place. Energy balancing cupping can help improve energy flow, restore balance, and support overall vitality.

Remember to follow proper safety guidelines and consult with a qualified cupping therapy practitioner before practicing self-care cupping techniques. They can provide guidance on cup selection, proper technique, and any precautions specific to your needs.

Incorporating self-care cupping techniques into your routine can be a powerful way to enhance your overall well-being. Whether you choose facial cupping, back cupping, cellulite cupping, reflexology cupping, or energy balancing cupping, these techniques offer a convenient and effective means to experience the therapeutic benefits of cupping therapy in the comfort of your own home.

Chapter Forty-Five

Cupping Therapy at Home

Cupping therapy, once exclusively performed in clinical settings, can now be practiced in the comfort of your own home. With the availability of at-home cupping kits and proper knowledge of the techniques involved, individuals can enjoy the benefits of cupping therapy without the need for a professional practitioner. Let's explore how cupping therapy can be safely and effectively practiced at home.

Choosing the Right Cupping Kit: The first step in practicing cupping therapy at home is to choose the right cupping kit. There are various types of cupping kits available, including silicone cups, suction cups, and fire cups. Consider your comfort level, desired treatment areas, and specific needs when selecting a kit. It's important to opt for high-quality cups that are safe, easy to use, and appropriate for self-application.

Familiarize Yourself with Cupping Techniques: Before starting your at-home cupping therapy, it's crucial to familiarize yourself with the different cupping techniques. These techniques include stationary cupping, sliding cupping, flash cupping, and pumping cupping. Each technique has its own benefits and application method. Take the time to learn and understand these techniques to ensure a safe and effective practice.

Preparing the Treatment Area: Creating a suitable environment for your cupping therapy session is important. Ensure that the treatment area is clean, well-lit, and comfortable. Consider using a towel or mat to provide cushioning and prevent the cups from slipping during the session. Additionally, make sure to remove any objects or obstacles that could interfere with your session.

Applying Cupping Techniques: Once you are familiar with the cupping techniques, you can apply them to your chosen treatment areas. Start by applying a thin layer of oil or lubricant to the skin to create a smooth surface for cup application. Follow the instructions provided with your cupping kit to create the desired suction. For stationary cupping, place the cup on the skin and leave it in place for the recommended duration. For sliding cupping, glide the cup over the skin using gentle, controlled movements.

Monitoring the Session: It's important to be mindful and monitor your cupping therapy session. Pay attention to the sensations you experience during the treatment, such as the level of suction, warmth, or pulling sensations. If you feel any discomfort or excessive pain, immediately remove the cup and discontinue the session. Remember to start with shorter sessions and gradually increase the duration as you become more comfortable with the practice.

Post-Cupping Care: After completing your cupping therapy session, it's essential to practice proper post-care. Gently remove the cups by breaking the seal, and avoid dragging them across the skin. Apply a moisturizer or healing balm to the treated areas to nourish and protect the skin. Hydrate your body by drinking water and engaging in light stretching exercises to promote circulation and aid in the body's natural healing process.

Educate Yourself: Continuously educate yourself on cupping therapy techniques and safety precautions. Stay updated with reliable sources, research studies, and reputable practitioners. Attend workshops or seek guidance from qualified cupping therapy professionals to enhance your knowledge and skills.

While practicing cupping therapy at home can be a beneficial self-care practice, it's important to note that certain conditions may require professional guidance. If you have any underlying health concerns, are pregnant, or have specific treatment needs, it is advisable to consult with a qualified cupping therapy practitioner before attempting at-home sessions.

Chapter Forty-Six

Cupping Therapy and Essential Oils

Cupping therapy and essential oils are two complementary practices that can be combined to enhance the therapeutic benefits of both modalities. Essential oils are highly concentrated plant extracts known for their aromatic and therapeutic properties. When used in conjunction with cupping therapy, essential oils can amplify the overall healing experience. Let's explore the relationship between cupping therapy and essential oils.

Choosing the Right Essential Oils: The selection of essential oils is a crucial step in combining them with cupping therapy. Different essential oils have unique properties and benefits. For example, lavender oil is known for its calming and relaxing effects, while peppermint oil has invigorating and refreshing properties. Consider your specific needs and goals when choosing the essential oils that will complement your cupping therapy session.

Pre-Cupping Oil Application: Before applying the cups, it is common to apply a thin layer of oil to the skin. This not only helps create a smooth surface for cup gliding but also allows the essential oils to be absorbed by the skin. Dilute the essential oil of your choice in a carrier oil, such as jojoba or coconut oil, and apply it to the treatment area. The combination of cupping therapy and essential oils can enhance the overall experience and promote relaxation and well-being.

Aromatherapy Diffusion: In addition to applying essential oils topically, aromatherapy diffusion can also be incorporated into your cupping therapy session. Diffusing essential oils into the air creates a pleasant and therapeutic atmosphere. Use an essential oil diffuser or simply add a few drops of your chosen essential oil to a bowl of hot water and inhale the aromatic vapors during the session. This can enhance relaxation, promote deep breathing, and complement the effects of cupping therapy.

Custom Blends for Specific Needs: Essential oils can be blended to target specific concerns or conditions. For example, if you are seeking relief from muscle soreness, you can create a blend of lavender, eucalyptus, and marjoram oils known for their analgesic and anti-inflammatory properties. Consult reliable resources, such as aromatherapy books or practitioners, to create custom blends that address your unique needs and preferences.

Post-Cupping Oil Application: After completing your cupping therapy session, you can continue to reap the benefits of essential oils by applying them to the treated areas. Dilute your chosen essential oil in a carrier oil and gently massage it into the skin. This can help nourish the skin, promote relaxation, and support the body's healing process.

Safety Precautions: While essential oils can be beneficial, it is important to exercise caution and follow safety guidelines. Essential oils are potent substances and should be used in appropriate dilutions. Conduct a patch test before applying essential oils to the skin to ensure you do not have any adverse reactions. If you have sensitive skin or underlying health conditions, consult with a qualified aromatherapist or healthcare professional for guidance on using essential oils safely.

Personal Preferences and Sensitivities: Each individual may have different preferences and sensitivities when it comes to essential oils. Some people may be more sensitive to certain scents or specific essential oil components.

Listen to your body and adjust your essential oil choices accordingly. If you experience any discomfort or irritation, discontinue use and seek professional advice.

Chapter Forty-Seven

Cupping Therapy and Other Alternative Therapies

Cupping therapy is often combined with other alternative therapies to create a holistic approach to wellness and healing. These therapies can complement cupping therapy by addressing various aspects of the body and mind, promoting balance, and supporting overall well-being. Let's explore some popular alternative therapies that can be integrated with cupping therapy.

Acupuncture: Acupuncture is an ancient Chinese healing practice that involves inserting thin needles into specific points on the body. Cupping therapy and acupuncture are often used together to enhance the effects of each modality. The combination of cupping and acupuncture can help balance energy flow, relieve pain, and promote overall health and wellness.

Massage Therapy: Massage therapy and cupping therapy work synergistically to provide a comprehensive approach to relaxation and healing. Massage techniques, such as Swedish massage, deep tissue massage, or myofascial release, can be incorporated before or after cupping therapy sessions. Massage helps relax muscles, improve circulation, and release tension, while cupping therapy targets specific areas of concern and promotes detoxification.

Herbal Medicine: Herbal medicine involves the use of plant-based remedies to support healing and promote well-being. Integrating cupping therapy with herbal medicine can provide a comprehensive approach to addressing specific health concerns. Herbal formulas or topical applications can be used in conjunction with cupping therapy to enhance the therapeutic effects and support the body's natural healing processes.

Meditation and Mindfulness: Cupping therapy can be combined with meditation and mindfulness practices to create a holistic approach to mental and emotional well-being. Engaging in mindfulness meditation before or after cupping therapy sessions helps calm the mind, reduce stress, and enhance relaxation. Practicing mindfulness during cupping therapy sessions allows for a deeper connection with the body and enhances the overall therapeutic experience.

Yoga and Stretching: Integrating cupping therapy with yoga and stretching exercises can promote flexibility, release tension, and improve overall physical well-being. Before or after cupping therapy, engage in gentle yoga poses or stretching routines that target areas of concern. Yoga and stretching complement cupping therapy by promoting circulation, enhancing range of motion, and supporting overall balance and flexibility.

Reiki: Reiki is an energy healing practice that involves the gentle laying on of hands to promote balance and well-being. Combining cupping therapy with Reiki can enhance the energetic aspect of the treatment. Reiki practitioners can incorporate their healing energy into the cupping therapy session, providing an additional layer of relaxation and support.

Chiropractic Care: Cupping therapy can be integrated with chiropractic care to provide a comprehensive approach to musculoskeletal health. Chiropractic adjustments, along with cupping therapy, can help relieve pain, improve spinal alignment, and enhance overall mobility and function.

It's important to note that while combining cupping therapy with other alternative therapies can offer numerous benefits, it is crucial to consult with qualified practitioners in each respective modality. These practitioners can provide guidance and create an individualized treatment plan based on your specific needs and goals.

Chapter Forty-Eight

Acupuncture and Cupping Therapy

Acupuncture and cupping therapy are two ancient healing modalities rooted in Traditional Chinese Medicine (TCM). While they can be practiced individually, they are often combined to create a synergistic and holistic approach to healing and well-being. Let's explore the relationship between acupuncture and cupping therapy and how they complement each other.

Acupuncture is a technique that involves inserting thin needles into specific points on the body. These points are believed to be interconnected along pathways called meridians, which correspond to different organs and systems in the body. The goal of acupuncture is to restore the balance of Qi, the vital life force, and promote the body's natural healing abilities.

Cupping therapy, on the other hand, involves creating a suction effect on the skin using cups. The cups can be made of various materials such as glass, silicone, or bamboo. This suction stimulates blood circulation, promotes lymphatic drainage, and helps release tension and toxins from the muscles and tissues.

When acupuncture and cupping therapy are combined, they work together to enhance the therapeutic effects. Here's how:

Balancing Energy: Acupuncture is known for its ability to balance the flow of energy in the body. By stimulating specific acupuncture points along the meridians, blockages or imbalances in the energy flow can be addressed.

Cupping therapy, with its ability to improve blood circulation and Qi flow, complements acupuncture by further enhancing the balance and harmony of energy within the body.

Targeted Treatment: Acupuncture and cupping therapy can be used together to address specific health concerns. Acupuncture needles are inserted into precise points based on the individual's condition, while cupping therapy can be applied to larger areas or specific muscle groups. This targeted approach allows for a comprehensive and tailored treatment plan to address both the underlying imbalances and the physical manifestations of the condition.

Pain Relief: Both acupuncture and cupping therapy are effective in relieving pain. Acupuncture needles stimulate the nervous system, releasing endorphins and other natural pain-relieving chemicals in the body. Cupping therapy helps to relax muscles, improve blood circulation, and alleviate muscle tension. When combined, they offer a powerful approach to pain management, providing relief for conditions such as chronic pain, muscle soreness, and sports injuries.

Detoxification: Cupping therapy is known for its ability to promote detoxification by improving blood and lymphatic circulation. The suction created by the cups helps to draw out toxins and metabolic waste from the tissues. When combined with acupuncture, which promotes the flow of Qi and removes energy blockages, the body's detoxification process is further supported.

Relaxation and Stress Reduction: Both acupuncture and cupping therapy have a deeply relaxing effect on the body and mind. Acupuncture helps to calm the nervous system, reduce stress, and promote a sense of well-being. Cupping therapy, with its gentle suction and release, induces a state of deep relaxation. When used together, they create a harmonious and soothing experience that helps reduce anxiety, improve sleep, and enhance overall relaxation.

It's important to note that acupuncture and cupping therapy should be performed by qualified and experienced practitioners. They will assess your individual condition, tailor the treatment plan to your needs, and ensure the safety and effectiveness of the combined therapy.

Chapter Forty-Nine

Cupping Therapy and Massage

Cupping therapy and massage are two therapeutic practices that can be combined to create a unique and effective approach to healing and relaxation. While they are distinct modalities, their integration can enhance the benefits of each technique. Let's explore the relationship between cupping therapy and massage and how they complement each other.

Cupping therapy involves creating suction on the skin using cups made of various materials, such as glass, silicone, or bamboo. This suction promotes blood circulation, releases muscle tension, and helps remove toxins from the body. On the other hand, massage therapy involves manual manipulation of the soft tissues to promote relaxation, relieve muscle tension, and improve overall well-being.

When cupping therapy and massage are combined, they work together synergistically to provide a comprehensive and deeply therapeutic experience. Here's how they complement each other:

Increased Circulation and Tissue Mobilization: Both cupping therapy and massage promote blood circulation and tissue mobilization. Cupping therapy enhances circulation by creating suction and drawing fresh blood to the treated areas. Massage, through manual manipulation, helps to break up adhesions and knots, improving circulation and releasing tension in the muscles. When used together, cupping therapy and massage enhance blood flow, allowing oxygen and nutrients to reach the tissues more efficiently, while simultaneously helping to relieve muscle tightness and promote relaxation.

Deeper Muscle Release: Cupping therapy and massage both target muscle tension, but they approach it from different angles. Cupping therapy uses suction to lift and stretch the underlying tissues, while massage uses various techniques such as kneading, compression, and stretching to release muscle knots and tightness. By combining cupping therapy with massage, the therapist can effectively address deep-seated muscle tension, trigger points, and adhesions, providing a more comprehensive and thorough release of muscle tension.

Enhanced Relaxation and Stress Reduction: Cupping therapy and massage have a profound effect on relaxation and stress reduction. Cupping therapy induces a sense of relaxation through the gentle suction and release, while massage therapy helps to calm the nervous system and promote the release of endorphins, the body's natural feel-good chemicals. When combined, cupping therapy and massage create a deeply relaxing experience, allowing for a greater sense of tranquility, stress relief, and overall well-being.

Detoxification: Cupping therapy is known for its ability to promote detoxification by improving lymphatic circulation and aiding in the removal of metabolic waste and toxins from the body. Massage, through its techniques and increased circulation, can also assist in the elimination of toxins. By integrating cupping therapy and massage, the body's detoxification process is supported on multiple levels, enhancing the elimination of waste and promoting overall detoxification.

Personalized Treatment: Cupping therapy and massage can be tailored to address specific needs and concerns. Each individual has unique areas of tension, discomfort, or specific goals for their treatment. By combining cupping therapy with massage, the therapist can create a personalized treatment plan that addresses the individual's specific needs. Cupping therapy can be applied to specific areas of concern before or after massage, providing targeted therapeutic benefits and promoting overall healing and relaxation.

It's important to note that cupping therapy and massage should be performed by qualified and experienced practitioners who understand the techniques and safety considerations associated with each modality. They will assess your individual condition, listen to your concerns, and create a treatment plan that integrates cupping therapy and massage to address your specific needs effectively.

Chapter Fifty

Cupping Therapy and Chiropractic Care

Cupping therapy and chiropractic care are two complementary approaches to health and wellness that can be combined to provide a comprehensive and holistic treatment plan. Both modalities aim to promote optimal function, restore balance, and alleviate pain or discomfort in the body. Let's explore the relationship between cupping therapy and chiropractic care and how they work together to support overall well-being.

Chiropractic care is a healthcare discipline that focuses on the diagnosis, treatment, and prevention of mechanical disorders of the musculoskeletal system, particularly the spine. Chiropractors use manual techniques, such as spinal adjustments, to restore proper alignment and function of the spine and other joints in the body. By doing so, they aim to relieve pain, improve mobility, and support the body's natural healing processes.

Cupping therapy, on the other hand, involves the application of suction cups to the skin, creating a vacuum effect. This suction promotes blood flow, releases muscle tension, and helps remove toxins and metabolic waste from the tissues. Cupping therapy can be used to address specific areas of concern or as a complementary treatment to support the overall chiropractic care plan.

When cupping therapy and chiropractic care are combined, they offer several benefits:

Enhanced Muscle Relaxation: Cupping therapy can be used to relax tight muscles and release trigger points, preparing the body for chiropractic adjustments. By reducing muscle tension and promoting relaxation, cupping therapy allows the chiropractor to perform adjustments more effectively and with greater ease. The combination of cupping therapy and chiropractic care supports the overall goal of relieving muscle tension and restoring proper function to the musculoskeletal system.

Improved Circulation: Cupping therapy increases blood circulation to the treated areas, which can aid in the healing process. Improved circulation helps deliver oxygen and nutrients to the tissues, while also removing metabolic waste and toxins. By enhancing circulation, cupping therapy supports the body's ability to heal and recover, allowing the chiropractic adjustments to have a greater impact.

Complementary Approach to Pain Relief: Cupping therapy and chiropractic care can work synergistically to provide pain relief. Cupping therapy helps alleviate muscle soreness, tension, and trigger points, while chiropractic adjustments address misalignments and joint dysfunctions that may contribute to pain. By combining these modalities, a comprehensive approach to pain management is achieved, targeting both the muscular and skeletal components of the pain experience.

Support for Recovery and Rehabilitation: Cupping therapy can be beneficial in supporting the recovery and rehabilitation process following chiropractic adjustments or other treatments. It can help reduce inflammation, increase range of motion, and promote tissue healing. By integrating cupping therapy into a chiropractic care plan, patients may experience accelerated recovery and improved overall outcomes.

Holistic Approach to Well-being: The combination of cupping therapy and chiropractic care promotes a holistic approach to well-being. Chiropractic care focuses on the alignment and function of the spine and nervous system, while cupping therapy targets the soft tissues and promotes overall circulation and relaxation. By addressing multiple aspects of health, these modalities work together to support the body's natural healing mechanisms and promote overall wellness.

It's important to consult with qualified professionals in both cupping therapy and chiropractic care to ensure safe and effective integration of the two modalities. They will assess your individual condition, consider your specific needs, and create a personalized treatment plan that incorporates cupping therapy and chiropractic adjustments to address your unique concerns and goals.

Chapter Fifty-One

Cupping Therapy and the Future

Cupping therapy, an ancient healing practice rooted in Traditional Chinese Medicine (TCM), has gained widespread recognition and popularity in recent years. As more people seek alternative and holistic approaches to health and well-being, cupping therapy has emerged as a viable option. Looking ahead, the future of cupping therapy holds promising potential for further integration and advancements. Let's explore some aspects that illustrate how cupping therapy is evolving and shaping the future of healthcare.

Research and Scientific Validation: As interest in cupping therapy grows, there is a greater emphasis on conducting scientific research to validate its effectiveness and understand its mechanisms of action. Researchers are investigating the physiological and biochemical responses associated with cupping therapy, exploring its effects on circulation, pain management, inflammation, and more. Scientific validation will provide a solid foundation for integrating cupping therapy into conventional healthcare settings and expand its acceptance among medical professionals.

Technology and Innovation: Technological advancements are paving the way for new cupping therapy techniques and tools. Innovations in cupping equipment, such as the development of adjustable suction cups, programmable cupping devices, and even wearable cupping technology, are being explored. These advancements aim to enhance the effectiveness, efficiency, and convenience of cupping therapy, making it more accessible to a wider range of individuals.

Integration with Digital Platforms: The digital age has opened up new possibilities for the integration of cupping therapy into digital platforms. Mobile applications and online platforms can provide educational resources, instructional videos, and virtual consultations with cupping therapy practitioners. These digital tools can help individuals learn about cupping therapy, find qualified practitioners, and access support and guidance throughout their cupping therapy journey.

Holistic Healthcare Practices: Cupping therapy aligns with the growing interest in holistic approaches to healthcare. As people seek comprehensive and integrative approaches that address the mind, body, and spirit, cupping therapy fits into the larger framework of holistic healing. In the future, we can expect to see cupping therapy being integrated into more holistic healthcare practices, alongside modalities such as acupuncture, massage therapy, nutrition, and mindfulness.

Personalized Treatment Plans: With the recognition of individual differences and the concept of personalized medicine, cupping therapy can be tailored to suit the unique needs of each individual. Cupping therapy practitioners can customize treatment plans based on factors such as medical history, specific health concerns, and lifestyle considerations. This personalized approach ensures that individuals receive the most effective and relevant cupping therapy for their specific needs, optimizing outcomes and patient satisfaction.

Collaboration with Conventional Medicine: The future of cupping therapy also lies in its collaboration with conventional medicine. As awareness and understanding of cupping therapy increase, medical professionals may incorporate it as an adjunct therapy in conventional treatment plans.

Cupping therapy can complement conventional medicine by providing additional support in pain management, stress reduction, rehabilitation, and overall wellness.

Education and Professional Standards: With the growing interest in cupping therapy, there is an increased emphasis on professional standards and education. Accredited training programs, certifications, and continuing education opportunities for cupping therapy practitioners are becoming more prevalent. This ensures that practitioners adhere to safe and ethical practices while providing quality care to individuals seeking cupping therapy.

Chapter Fifty-Two

Research on Cupping Therapy

Research on cupping therapy, an ancient healing practice that involves creating suction on the skin using cups, has gained momentum in recent years. As the popularity of cupping therapy continues to rise, scientists and researchers are exploring its effectiveness, safety, and underlying mechanisms. Let's delve into the research on cupping therapy and highlight some key findings.

Pain Management: Several studies have investigated the efficacy of cupping therapy in managing various types of pain, including musculoskeletal pain, back pain, neck pain, and migraine headaches. Research suggests that cupping therapy can provide significant pain relief by reducing muscle tension, improving blood circulation, and activating the body's natural pain modulation mechanisms.

Inflammatory Conditions: Cupping therapy has been studied for its potential anti-inflammatory effects. Research indicates that cupping therapy may help reduce inflammation by stimulating the release of anti-inflammatory cytokines, promoting blood flow, and enhancing the activity of immune cells involved in the inflammatory response. This makes cupping therapy a potential adjunct therapy for inflammatory conditions such as arthritis, asthma, and inflammatory bowel disease.

Blood Circulation and Microcirculation: Cupping therapy has been shown to improve blood circulation and microcirculation. Studies using various imaging techniques have demonstrated increased blood flow and oxygenation in the treated areas. This enhanced circulation can support tissue healing, nutrient delivery, and waste removal, contributing to overall health and well-being.

Psychological and Emotional Well-being: Research suggests that cupping therapy may have positive effects on psychological and emotional well-being. It has been shown to reduce anxiety, stress, and depression symptoms, promoting a sense of relaxation and improved mood. Cupping therapy may achieve these effects through its ability to induce physical relaxation, stimulate the release of endorphins, and regulate the autonomic nervous system.

Dermatological Conditions: Cupping therapy has been explored for its potential benefits in various dermatological conditions. Research indicates its efficacy in reducing symptoms of acne, eczema, and herpes zoster. Cupping therapy may improve these conditions by enhancing local blood circulation, reducing inflammation, and promoting tissue regeneration.

Safety and Adverse Effects: Studies have evaluated the safety of cupping therapy and reported minimal adverse effects. Common side effects include temporary skin discoloration, mild discomfort, and the formation of circular marks or bruises. Serious complications are rare when cupping therapy is performed by trained professionals using appropriate techniques and precautions.

Mechanisms of Action: Researchers have sought to understand the underlying mechanisms of cupping therapy. Studies have shown that cupping therapy affects various physiological processes, including sensory stimulation, nerve reflexes, immune responses, and connective tissue remodeling. These mechanisms contribute to the therapeutic effects observed in cupping therapy.

Comparison Studies: Some studies have compared cupping therapy with other interventions or control groups. For example, research has compared cupping therapy with conventional treatments, such as medication or physical therapy, and alternative therapies, such as acupuncture or herbal medicine. These comparison studies help provide insights into the relative efficacy and unique contributions of cupping therapy in specific conditions.

Chapter Fifty-Three

Advancements in Cupping Therapy

Advancements in cupping therapy have been occurring at a rapid pace, driven by increased interest, research, and innovation in the field. This ancient healing practice, rooted in Traditional Chinese Medicine, has evolved over time to meet the needs of modern healthcare. Let's explore some of the noteworthy advancements in cupping therapy that have contributed to its continued growth and integration into contemporary practice.

Improved Cupping Equipment: The development of new and improved cupping equipment has significantly enhanced the practice of cupping therapy. Traditional glass cups have been supplemented by modern materials such as silicone, plastic, and bamboo. These materials offer advantages such as durability, flexibility, and ease of use. Furthermore, adjustable suction cups, which allow for precise control of the suction strength, have been introduced, enhancing the safety and effectiveness of cupping therapy.

Cupping Techniques: Advancements in cupping techniques have expanded the range of treatment options available. Alongside traditional stationary cupping, dynamic cupping techniques have gained popularity. This involves moving the cups along the body surface, either manually or with the help of mechanical devices. Dynamic cupping allows for a broader coverage of the affected areas and provides a different sensory experience for the patient.

Integration with Technology: Cupping therapy has embraced technological advancements to enhance its practice. Electronic cupping devices, which use air pressure or suction control mechanisms, provide a consistent and controlled therapeutic experience. Additionally, wearable cupping technology, such as silicone cups with embedded magnets or pressure points, allows individuals to receive continuous treatment and self-care outside of traditional clinic settings.

Combination Therapies: Cupping therapy has been increasingly integrated with other complementary therapies to create synergistic treatment approaches. For example, cupping therapy is often combined with acupuncture, massage therapy, or chiropractic adjustments to enhance the therapeutic effects. These integrative approaches offer a more comprehensive and tailored treatment plan, addressing multiple aspects of health and well-being.

Research and Evidence Base: The growing body of research on cupping therapy has contributed to its advancement and acceptance in the medical community. Scientific studies have investigated the physiological and psychological effects of cupping therapy, its efficacy in various conditions, and its safety profile. The accumulation of evidence supports the integration of cupping therapy into clinical practice and provides a foundation for further exploration and refinement.

Standardization and Professional Guidelines: Efforts have been made to establish standardized practices and guidelines for cupping therapy. Professional organizations and regulatory bodies have developed codes of conduct, training requirements, and safety protocols to ensure the ethical and safe practice of cupping therapy. These standards promote consistency, professionalism, and patient safety across practitioners and enhance the credibility of cupping therapy as a legitimate healthcare modality.

Education and Training: The availability of comprehensive education and training programs has expanded, equipping practitioners with the knowledge and skills required for safe and effective cupping therapy practice. Accredited courses, workshops, and continuing education opportunities allow practitioners to stay updated on the latest advancements, techniques, and research in cupping therapy. This ongoing professional development ensures the delivery of high-quality care to individuals seeking cupping therapy.

Integration into Mainstream Healthcare: Advancements in cupping therapy have contributed to its integration into mainstream healthcare settings. Increasingly, medical professionals, such as physicians, physical therapists, and nurses, are incorporating cupping therapy into their treatment plans. This integration allows for a collaborative and multidisciplinary approach to patient care, where cupping therapy can complement conventional interventions and enhance patient outcomes.

Chapter Fifty-Four

Integrating Cupping Therapy into Mainstream Healthcare

Integrating cupping therapy into mainstream healthcare represents a significant shift in the way traditional healing practices are viewed and utilized. Cupping therapy, rooted in ancient healing traditions, has gained recognition for its therapeutic benefits and is increasingly being integrated into conventional healthcare settings. Let's explore the reasons behind this integration and the potential benefits it offers.

Expanding Treatment Options: Integrating cupping therapy into mainstream healthcare expands the range of treatment options available to patients. Traditional medical approaches often focus on pharmacological interventions or surgical procedures. By incorporating cupping therapy, healthcare providers can offer a non-invasive and drug-free alternative for managing various conditions. This integrative approach allows for a more personalized and comprehensive treatment plan, catering to individual needs and preferences.

Addressing Holistic Well-being: Cupping therapy aligns with the growing recognition of the importance of holistic well-being. It recognizes the interconnectedness of the mind, body, and spirit and acknowledges the impact of emotional and energetic factors on health. Integrating cupping therapy into mainstream healthcare acknowledges the importance of addressing not only physical symptoms but also psychological and emotional aspects of health. This holistic approach can enhance patient outcomes and overall well-being.

Supporting Patient-Centered Care: Integrating cupping therapy promotes patient-centered care, focusing on the individual's needs, preferences, and goals. It empowers patients by providing them with choices and involving them in the decision-making process. By offering cupping therapy as a treatment option, healthcare providers acknowledge the value of patient perspectives and provide a more inclusive and personalized approach to healthcare.

Complementing Conventional Treatments: Cupping therapy can complement conventional medical treatments, enhancing their effectiveness and promoting holistic healing. For example, cupping therapy can be integrated into pain management protocols to reduce reliance on pain medications or used alongside physical therapy to improve outcomes. By combining traditional and conventional approaches, healthcare providers can optimize patient care and achieve better outcomes.

Supporting Preventive Healthcare: Integrating cupping therapy into mainstream healthcare can also support preventive healthcare strategies. Cupping therapy, when used proactively, can help maintain overall well-being, improve circulation, release muscle tension, and enhance the body's natural healing processes. Incorporating cupping therapy into routine healthcare visits can help individuals prevent the development of chronic conditions and promote long-term wellness.

Evidenced-Based Practice: The growing body of scientific research on cupping therapy provides a foundation for its integration into mainstream healthcare. Evidence-based practice relies on research findings to guide clinical decisions and ensure the effectiveness and safety of interventions. With increasing research supporting the therapeutic benefits of cupping therapy, healthcare providers can confidently incorporate it into their practice, knowing that it is grounded in scientific evidence.

Collaboration and Multidisciplinary Care: Integrating cupping therapy fosters collaboration and multidisciplinary care. Healthcare providers from different disciplines, such as physicians, physical therapists, acupuncturists, and massage therapists, can work together to develop comprehensive treatment plans that address the diverse needs of patients. This collaboration allows for a synergistic approach, combining the strengths of various modalities to optimize patient outcomes.

Patient Satisfaction and Well-being: Integrating cupping therapy into mainstream healthcare can contribute to increased patient satisfaction and well-being. Cupping therapy often provides a unique and relaxing experience for patients, promoting a sense of well-being and improved quality of life. Patients appreciate having access to diverse treatment options and being actively involved in their healthcare decisions, leading to higher levels of satisfaction and engagement in their own healing journey.

Chapter Fifty-Five

The Benefits of Cupping Therapy

Cupping therapy, an ancient healing practice with roots in Traditional Chinese Medicine, has gained recognition for its numerous therapeutic benefits. This non-invasive technique involves creating suction on the skin to promote healing, relaxation, and overall well-being. Let's explore some of the key benefits of cupping therapy and how it can positively impact physical and mental health.

Pain Relief: Cupping therapy is widely used for pain management. The suction created by the cups helps increase blood circulation to the affected area, promoting the delivery of oxygen and nutrients while removing metabolic waste. This increased blood flow can relieve muscle tension, reduce inflammation, and alleviate pain caused by conditions such as musculoskeletal disorders, migraines, and fibromyalgia.

Improved Blood Circulation: Cupping therapy enhances blood circulation and microcirculation. By drawing blood to the surface of the skin, cupping stimulates the expansion of blood vessels, promoting better blood flow throughout the body. Improved circulation not only benefits the musculoskeletal system but also supports overall health, aiding in the delivery of nutrients, removal of toxins, and optimal organ function.

Reduced Inflammation: Inflammation is a common underlying factor in various health conditions. Cupping therapy has been found to have anti-inflammatory effects by triggering the release of anti-inflammatory substances and modulating the immune response. It can help alleviate symptoms associated with conditions such as arthritis, asthma, allergies, and autoimmune disorders.

Relaxation and Stress Reduction: Cupping therapy promotes relaxation and helps reduce stress. The gentle suction of the cups creates a sensation of deep relaxation, triggering the parasympathetic nervous system response, often referred to as the "rest and digest" mode. This response promotes a sense of calmness, relieves anxiety, and aids in stress management.

Detoxification: Cupping therapy can support the body's natural detoxification processes. The suction created by the cups helps to draw out toxins and metabolic waste from the tissues, assisting the lymphatic system in flushing them out of the body. This detoxifying effect can help improve overall cellular function and support the body's natural healing and rejuvenation processes.

Enhanced Sports Performance and Recovery: Cupping therapy is increasingly utilized by athletes and fitness enthusiasts to enhance sports performance and aid in recovery. By promoting blood circulation, it can help increase oxygenation and nutrient supply to muscles, reducing post-exercise fatigue and promoting faster recovery. Additionally, cupping therapy can help alleviate muscle soreness and improve flexibility, contributing to improved athletic performance.

Skin Health and Beauty: Cupping therapy has benefits for skin health and beauty. By increasing blood flow to the skin, it promotes nourishment and rejuvenation, aiding in the reduction of fine lines, wrinkles, and cellulite. Cupping therapy can also improve the appearance of scars, stretch marks, and acne by stimulating collagen production and tissue regeneration.

Respiratory Health: Cupping therapy is often used to alleviate respiratory symptoms and promote lung health. It can help loosen mucus and congestion, making it easier to breathe. Cupping therapy is commonly applied to the upper back and chest to target respiratory conditions such as asthma, bronchitis, and common colds.

Balancing Energy and Qi: According to Traditional Chinese Medicine, cupping therapy helps balance the flow of energy, or Qi, in the body. By targeting specific acupoints and meridians, cupping therapy aims to restore the harmonious flow of energy, promoting overall health and well-being.

Chapter Fifty-Six

The Future of Cupping Therapy

The future of cupping therapy is promising, as this ancient healing practice continues to gain recognition and acceptance in both traditional and modern healthcare settings. With ongoing research, technological advancements, and an increased focus on holistic well-being, cupping therapy is poised to play an even greater role in supporting overall health and wellness. Let's explore some key areas that shape the future of cupping therapy.

Research Advancements: Research on cupping therapy is expanding, shedding light on its mechanisms of action, efficacy, and safety. Continued scientific inquiry will help build a robust evidence base for cupping therapy, providing healthcare providers with more comprehensive information to guide treatment decisions. Further research may explore its effects on specific conditions, optimal treatment protocols, and long-term outcomes.

Integration into Mainstream Healthcare: Cupping therapy is gradually being integrated into mainstream healthcare systems. As more healthcare providers recognize its benefits and evidence-based support, they are incorporating cupping therapy into their treatment offerings. This integration will continue to promote collaboration between traditional and conventional healthcare approaches, resulting in more comprehensive and personalized patient care.

Technology and Innovation: Technological advancements have the potential to enhance the practice of cupping therapy. New tools and devices, such as electronic or automated cupping devices, can provide precise control over suction and offer consistent treatment experiences. Additionally, the integration of digital health platforms may facilitate remote monitoring, personalized treatment plans, and improved patient outcomes.

Customized Treatment Approaches: The future of cupping therapy will likely involve a more individualized and tailored approach. Healthcare providers may combine cupping therapy with other modalities, such as acupuncture, massage, or physical therapy, to create personalized treatment plans based on a patient's specific needs and goals. This holistic and patient-centered approach will allow for better outcomes and increased patient satisfaction.

Education and Training: The importance of education and training in cupping therapy will continue to grow. Accredited programs and courses will be developed to ensure practitioners receive comprehensive training, emphasizing safe and effective cupping techniques. Continued education and professional development opportunities will equip practitioners with the necessary skills and knowledge to deliver high-quality cupping therapy.

Standardization and Regulations: As cupping therapy becomes more widely accepted, efforts to establish standardization and regulations will likely increase. Professional organizations and regulatory bodies will work towards developing guidelines for safe practice, ethical conduct, and competency standards for cupping therapy practitioners. Standardization will promote consistency, quality assurance, and patient safety across different healthcare settings.

Public Awareness and Acceptance: The future of cupping therapy relies on increasing public awareness and acceptance. As individuals seek alternative and complementary approaches to health, cupping therapy's benefits will become more widely known. Media exposure, public education campaigns, and testimonials from satisfied patients will contribute to a greater understanding and acceptance of cupping therapy as a viable healthcare option.

Collaboration with Other Modalities: Cupping therapy will likely continue to collaborate with other complementary modalities to offer more comprehensive care. Integrative medicine approaches that combine cupping therapy with acupuncture, herbal medicine, nutritional counseling, or mindfulness practices can create synergistic effects and enhance overall treatment outcomes.

Chapter Fifty-Seven

Incorporating Cupping Therapy into Your Health and Wellness Routine.

Incorporating cupping therapy into your health and wellness routine can be a valuable addition to support your overall well-being. This ancient healing practice, rooted in Traditional Chinese Medicine, offers a range of benefits that can enhance your physical, mental, and emotional health. Let's explore some key considerations and tips for incorporating cupping therapy into your routine.

Consult with a Qualified Practitioner: Before beginning cupping therapy, it's essential to consult with a qualified and experienced practitioner. They can assess your health history, discuss your specific concerns, and determine if cupping therapy is appropriate for you. A trained practitioner will also ensure that the treatment is administered safely and effectively.

Set Clear Goals: Before starting cupping therapy, identify your specific health and wellness goals. Whether you seek pain relief, stress reduction, improved circulation, or general well-being, clearly defining your objectives will help guide your cupping therapy sessions and measure progress over time.

Incorporate Regular Sessions: Consistency is key when incorporating cupping therapy into your routine. Regular sessions allow for cumulative benefits and provide an opportunity for your body to respond and adapt to the treatment. Discuss with your practitioner the recommended frequency and duration of cupping sessions based on your individual needs.

Combine with Other Modalities: Cupping therapy can be complemented by other health and wellness practices. Consider integrating cupping therapy with activities such as yoga, meditation, acupuncture, or massage. This combination can create a synergistic effect, amplifying the benefits and promoting a holistic approach to your health and well-being.

Practice Self-Care: Cupping therapy can be extended beyond the treatment session through self-care practices. Self-administered cupping techniques, such as silicone or suction cups, can be incorporated into your daily routine to target specific areas of concern. This allows you to experience the benefits of cupping therapy between professional sessions and maintain continuity in your well-being journey.

Listen to Your Body: Pay attention to how your body responds to cupping therapy. Each person's experience may vary, so it's important to listen to your body's signals and communicate with your practitioner. If you experience any discomfort or adverse effects, inform your practitioner so that adjustments can be made to the treatment plan.

Hydrate and Rest: After a cupping therapy session, it's essential to stay hydrated and rest. Cupping therapy can stimulate circulation and release toxins, so drinking plenty of water can support the elimination of waste from your system. Resting allows your body to recover and optimize the benefits of the treatment.

Maintain Open Communication: Effective communication with your cupping therapy practitioner is crucial throughout your journey. Share any changes in your health status, concerns, or feedback regarding the treatment. Your practitioner can adjust the treatment plan accordingly to ensure that your needs are met and that you have a positive experience.

Educate Yourself: Take the time to educate yourself about cupping therapy. Read reputable sources, consult books, or explore reliable online resources to deepen your understanding of the practice. This knowledge will help you make informed decisions and actively participate in your health and wellness journey.

Monitor Progress: Keep track of your progress and the effects of cupping therapy on your overall well-being. Regularly assess whether your goals are being met, and make adjustments as needed. Monitoring your progress allows you to evaluate the effectiveness of cupping therapy and make informed decisions about its continued integration into your health and wellness routine.

Incorporating cupping therapy into your health and wellness routine can be a transformative experience. By following these tips and working with a qualified practitioner, you can maximize the benefits of cupping therapy and enhance your overall well-being.

SD - #0183 - 070926 - C0 - 229/152/9 - PB - 9781776968121 - Matt Lamination